STOP STUTTERING

Also by Dr. Martin F. Schwartz

Stuttering Solved

Stop Stuttering

DR. MARTIN F. SCHWARTZ

AND

DR. GRADY L. CARTER

Fitzhenry & Whiteside
Toronto, Ottawa, Halifax
Winnipeg, Edmonton
Vancouver

Grateful acknowledgment is made for permission to reprint the excerpt from *The Road Less Traveled* by M. Scott Peck, M.D., copyright © 1978 by M. Scott Peck, M.D. Reprinted by permission of Simon & Schuster, Inc.

Fitzhenry & Whiteside Limited
195 Allstate Parkway
Markham, Ontario L3R 4T8

Canadian Cataloguing in Publication Data

Schwartz, Martin F., 1936–
  Stop stuttering

ISBN 0-88902-919-9

1. Stuttering. 2. Stuttering—Case studies. 3. Stuttering—Patients—Biography—United States. 4. Carter, Grady L.—Health. I. Carter, Grady L. II. Title.

RC424.S37   1986   616.85'5406   C86-093334-2

Contents

STOP STUTTERING

I

THE METHOD

by Dr. Martin F. Schwartz

Acknowledgments

I wish to acknowledge all of those responsible for the writing of my portion of this book. My colleagues at the National Center for Stuttering for providing the structure within which a substantial clinical experience was obtained; my patients, who, with a knowledge of stuttering greater than mine, at all times gently guided me to new insights and understandings; and last, but certainly not least, to my wife, Judith, who provided encouragement and support throughout and enabled this work to be produced.

Introduction

In my first book, *Stuttering Solved,* I described a new treatment for stuttering based on my discovery of its physical cause. The 89 percent success rate reported with this new treatment provoked considerable interest among the stuttering and nonstuttering public. The interest, I discovered, was not only a response to the success rate, but also a reaction to the fact that I had demonstrated an entirely new cause of stuttering.

Much research has been published in the decade since. This research has brought about major changes in my basic understanding of the cause of stuttering and has significantly altered the techniques of treatment. Success rates now approach 100 percent.

Having successful techniques, however, and getting people to use them are two very different things. Oscar Wilde was once asked by a reporter if he thought his upcoming play would be a success. His response was, "My dear fellow, the play is a success; the question is, will the audience be one." And that response applies here as well. We now have a technique we know to be successful; the question is: why don't all stutterers learn it?

In this book Dr. Carter and I try to answer this question by taking the reader beyond an understanding of stuttering to a detailed description of the eventual transformation of a stutterer into a nonstutterer. In essence, we deal with the issue of recovery: the process by which a therapy is *absorbed* and through such absorption creates a new and lasting entity.

In my first book I knew very little about the process of change. I felt, somewhat naïvely, that if one were able to demonstrate to a group of reasonable, motivated, stuttering adults that here, for the first time, was a technique that absolutely worked, they would automatically use it.

Of course, I knew why previous therapies had failed; the answer was clear: the cause of stuttering had not been known. But things were different now, I felt. Here was a technique that was effective, easy to learn, and welcomed with no apparent resistance. Yet, for one reason or another, for one patient in nine, there was a failure to follow through.

Why did this happen? Were the patients lazy? Had they begun treatment against their will—at the urging of an anxious parent or committed spouse? Were they mentally incapable of processing the information? Were they afraid of fluency?

In the last ten years I have found the answers. I have become aware of the universe of things that can actively work to thwart attempts at change. Many of these things are conscious; many more are subconscious. But their impact is unmistakable. And they determine whether or not the audience will be a success.

My goal is to help people who stutter to stop their stuttering *permanently.* I know how to do this with any patient. Quite simply, if I were to employ my techniques with a stutterer *continuously* throughout the day and evening, reminding, encouraging, supporting, cajoling at all times, and the patient agreed to this arrangement, he* would be *permanently* fluent in a few months. It is frustrating to know this and know that the practical realities of

---

* The personal pronoun *he* shall be used throughout the book when referring to stutterers since approximately 80 percent of them are males.

day-to-day existence prohibit the very kind of relationship necessary to effect permanent changes in every stutterer.

So I often tell patients at the beginning of a workshop that I am going to treat them exactly as if they were therapists in training, that they are going to be treated as colleagues, not patients. I tell them that although they may be married or live in large families, ultimately it is they, and no one else, who live with themselves all of the time. And that if they are to make a permanent change, they must learn how to become their own therapist; ultimately, they must treat themselves.

I further tell them to imagine that there are two people within each of them, one a stutterer—frightened, withdrawn, frustrated—and the other an adult with whom we are communicating. I train the adult, and the adult must "parent" the frightened stutterer and guide him through the process of change.

Change requires courage, and courage on a sustained basis requires support, not only internal support, but external as well. Support groups of stutterers applying the techniques described in this book have been established in most major cities in the United States. Operating within a strict protocol, these group meetings motivate patients to dedicate themselves to practice, and provide a sympathetic audience during times of difficulty. The clubs share experiences through exchanges of tape cassettes, joint meetings, and the publication of a newsletter that provides inspiration, guidance, and practical information for dealing with a wide variety of difficult speaking situations.

Banquets are held every year throughout the United States. At these, through the mechanism of the after-dinner speech, patients celebrate their progress and successes. They talk about how their lives have changed, how their fears have evaporated, and about their incredible new sense of freedom to be able to say what they want to say, when they want to say it, where they want to say it. They are in control. They are no longer victims.

My portion of this book will describe what is new in the field of stuttering. It will enumerate the most recent refinements of the air-flow technique. It will outline the workshops that are the vehicles for learning these techniques. It will explain how the results of recent research into principles of general stress reduction have enhanced the original therapy, and how the discoveries of vitamin and mineral supplementation and nutrition are being successfully employed by a significant number of stutterers to expedite their attainment of fluency.

The book takes you from the workshop to the club meetings to refresher courses and finally to the banquets that are the final celebration of success.

The process of change takes time, typically a year or two. It is possible to learn in a day the techniques for producing fluency. Making a habit of them takes months. Using the habit to eradicate one's fears and change one's self-concept takes years. But it is a task well worth the effort.

DR. MARTIN F. SCHWARTZ

New York City, 1986

1

The Physical Basis
of Stuttering

The Myth of Stuttering as a Psychological Problem

Probably the most commonly held notion about stuttering is that it is a psychological problem. It is believed that stutterers have emotional problems or react badly under chronic, excessive stress. As an extreme example, in certain parts of India stutterers are viewed as possessed by demons, and are to be shunned lest the listener catch the contagion, especially if the listener is a child.

There is ample reason to accept a psychological explanation of stuttering. Stutterers acknowledge that their problems become worse under stress. They know that there are three specific fears to which they most often respond: the fear of certain words, certain sounds, and certain situations.

Stutterers know well in advance when they are going to stutter. They "see" the feared events. As a result, they often seek to avoid them, and since they are, as a group, intelligent (with an average IQ of 114), they soon become successful at these avoidance behaviors. Indeed, fully 20 percent of all stutterers never stutter. Rather, they situation-avoid and word-substitute. They will refuse a promotion if it involves making presentations before feared groups. They ask their spouses to make phone calls when telephoning is difficult for them (more than 80 percent of stutterers report telephoning to be one of their most troublesome speaking situations). Or they go into a restaurant and order only what they can say rather than what they want. And if they have trouble saying their name, which is a frequent occurrence, they either spell it or produce a business card.

There are about half a million of these hidden or "closet" stutterers in the United States. The price they pay for their hiding is high: continued vigilance whenever they speak. They must scan quickly for the feared words and be prepared to switch instantly even if what comes out is inaccurate, inappropriate, or even ludicrous.

It all seems to be a matter of stress. And stutterers for years have gone to psychologists and psychiatrists to have their problem treated. The reported results have not been encouraging. The stuttering has rarely, if ever, improved. And the usual explanation offered by the psychotherapist has been that the problem is so deep-seated, having most often begun somewhere between the ages of two and six, that it requires years of intensive therapy to get to its roots and handle it effectively.

One stutterer I saw had undergone seventeen years of psychotherapy at a total cost to date of approximately $85,000. I remember noting after my evaluation that this young man was probably the most well-adjusted stutterer I had ever seen.

To this very day, the mythology persists that stuttering is a psychological problem. Each year so-called experts write books that proclaim this fact loud and clear, and articles appear in both newspapers and magazines that reinforce this belief.

Psychiatrists continue to attempt to treat thousands of stutterers each year with techniques that have long since been proven inadequate. Freud knew they were inadequate. In one of his early works he wrote, "Whatever the source of stuttering is, it is not amenable to the treatments I have developed. I therefore refuse to attempt to deal with it further."

He was correct. And one wishes that his psychotherapist descendants would similarly acknowledge their inadequacy in this clinical area. But they persist, and a vast stuttering public seeks understanding through psychotherapy when, in fact, the physical cause has been known for a decade. Many stutterers are so persuaded that their problem is purely psychological that they absolutely, steadfastly refuse to participate in any other form of therapeutic enterprise, in spite of the fact that their stuttering is not improving.

I recall lecturing at a psychotherapy institute a number of years ago. In the audience were several stutterers who were also patients of two of the staff members at the institute. Encouraged by their therapists, they came to hear what I had to say about the subject and to review with me the research findings that supported my conclusions.

Several weeks later, I received a surreptitious phone call from one of them. He said he represented three stutterers who wanted to visit me as a group to hear more. But they didn't want the institute to know because they felt that such a visit would somehow demonstrate a breach of faith between them and their psychotherapists. And so would I mind keeping it to myself.

We met a short time thereafter one evening in a coffee shop. The meeting had a clandestine air about it. Here were three individuals who had stuttered all of their lives and who were attempting, with great trepidation, to admit that their lifelong belief systems about their problem were incorrect. Their desire to solve the problem was so great that it had overcome their reticence, and they were now seated with me asking a series of questions they had prepared.

One of the three eventually came for therapy. He was treated successfully, and several months later I asked him whether he had, since becoming fluent, seen his two colleagues. He reported that he saw them regularly at group psychotherapy meetings. I asked him about his speech at these meetings and he replied that it was perfect. I questioned him about the reaction of the other two to his fluency and his response was, "We never discuss it and of course I never told them that I came to see you."

Intrigued, I queried him further. "But why didn't you tell them?" And the answer was, "How could I? They thought the psychotherapy had worked for me. I was afraid that if they discovered that I wasn't stuttering because I had received a different form of treatment, I would not be able to handle revealing this to my therapists and to my stuttering colleagues. How could I justify my continued attendance at the group therapy meetings?"

The Physical Cause

In this book the first step is to dispel the mythology of the psychological cause by explaining the physical cause—describing it, showing how it was first discovered, and explaining how subsequent research has both refined and improved our understanding of it. Without an adequate understanding of stuttering it is impossible to understand why conventional therapies have failed and why the techniques described in the next chapters are so truly revolutionary.

If I were dealing with a patient in a clinical setting, I would insist that the patient have a complete understanding of the physical basis of his problem. Indeed, at workshops we go into great detail about the anatomy and physiology of the vocal cord area, since we have discovered that patients must be able to visualize the functioning of this area as they begin to practice the techniques that have been developed. At workshops, patients are even tested on the adequacy of their understanding, and great pains are taken to establish that, even for those as young as seven, a basic understanding is well rooted in the consciousness before proceeding.

Let us begin. Late in 1949, at a meeting held in Moscow at which representatives from all of the iron curtain countries were present, a decision was made to establish world supremacy in the Olympics as a demonstration of the superiority of Communist societies over "decadent" Western ones. A massive program was established, funded by each country, with a substantial amount of resource material, both in terms of personnel and money. Physiology laboratories were set up to specialize in the physiology of movement—specifically, movement related to sports. The results of these laboratory findings would be used to enhance athletic prowess in Olympic competition.

One laboratory, established in East Germany, was devoted to a study of the timing and strength of muscle activity during various sports. Electrodes were attached to different muscles to measure the muscle activity of champions in all major Olympic sports. Amateurs were similarly studied. The results enabled the East Germans to describe and to refine the muscular activities necessary for winning performances. Sports physiology had become a science.

One of the early findings showed that when individuals are placed under conditions of stress, they tense; that some tense more than others; and that they tend to focus tension in certain areas in their bodies. These focus areas were termed *targets*. Subsequent research demonstrated that targets varied considerably from individual to individual and that the three most common targets for human beings (laboratory animals had different targets) were the muscles of the abdominal wall, those of the shoulder girdle, and those of the face. It was found that 82 percent of all people possessed a target in one of these three areas. Targets were found to be congenital and frequently, but not always, inherited.

Knowledge of targets proved invaluable in the process of screening individuals for athletic training. For example, if, when placed under stress, an individual interested in becoming a world-class discus thrower tensed muscles that should be relaxed for an adequate performance in this sport, he was told that he would likely never reach world-class status in that activity and that he should select another, one that would be consistent with his congenital tensing patterns.

Surveys were made of all the muscles of the body and how they reacted under induced conditions of stress, and results were published in the mid-1950s. The reports showed that small groups of individuals had targets at their hands, lower back, and legs, and that a very small group had a target in and around the muscles of the vocal cords. Specifically, 2 percent of adults were born with a target at this area. *Subsequent research has shown that all stutterers come from this 2 percent subpopulation. That is, stutterers are born with a tendency, when under conditions of stress, to display an excessive degree of tensing within the muscles of their vocal cords.*

The vocal cords are two small horizontal folds of tissue that lie within the voice box, or larynx. The larynx rests on top of the trachea, or windpipe, and its front cover is the Adam's apple. Figure 1 on page 14 shows a drawing of these structures.

For someone to speak, the vocal cords are brought together by several pairs of muscles so that they lightly touch each other. The person then builds up air pressure beneath them by expelling air from the lungs. When the air pressure is great enough, it blows the vocal cords apart, setting them vibrating and making sound. This sound is the raw energy for speech production; it is converted into speech by moving the lips, tongue, jaw, teeth, palate, and other articulators.

With a stutterer this process is disrupted. Let us illustrate the details of this disruption by considering the onset of stuttering in a child. The typical child begins stuttering between the ages of two and six and has generally been speaking normally for a year or more. On a particular day, he is under some condition or conditions of stress. It is important to point out that what may be stressful for a three-year-old may not be stressful for an adult. A typical three-year-old's stress may be starting nursery school, moving to a new neighborhood, hearing his parents have an argument, or being left with grandma while his parents go on vacation. The important point is that the particular stress is *not* critical.

Since this child has been born with the tendency to target stress-

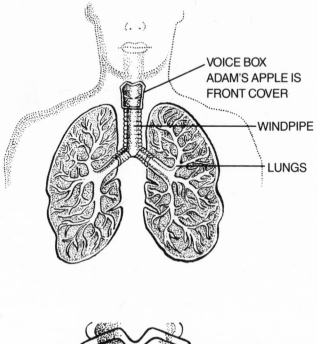

VOICE BOX
ADAM'S APPLE IS
FRONT COVER

WINDPIPE

LUNGS

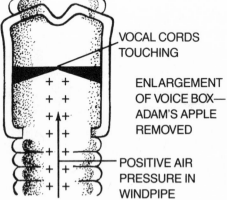

VOCAL CORDS
TOUCHING

ENLARGEMENT
OF VOICE BOX—
ADAM'S APPLE
REMOVED

POSITIVE AIR
PRESSURE IN
WINDPIPE

Figure 1   The vocal cords

induced tension at the muscles of the vocal cords, when the stress does occur and he attempts to speak, bringing his vocal cords together, the added tension causes his cords to suddenly lock. The technical term for the locking is a *laryngeal spasm.*

Suddenly, for the first time, the young child finds himself unable to speak. When this happens, he does something perfectly normal: he begins to struggle a bit to release the locked vocal cords. This struggle may appear at the lips and/or tongue and is called *primary stuttering.* It appears as seemingly effortless repetitions of words, sounds, or syllables, or hesitations. I use the word *seemingly* because these difficulties are not without effort but, rather, are low on the continuum of effort. The locking of the cords is not very great and the degree of struggle needed to release them is also not great.

An important characteristic of primary stuttering is that the young child is generally unaware of the fact that he is having difficulty. Only after a period of time does he become aware, either by directly hearing the difficulty himself or by observing the reactions of others. Once this happens he starts to become concerned, tenses even more, locks his cords tighter, and must intensify his struggle to release the lock. Now the struggler's behavior becomes forceful and moves into what therapists call *secondary stuttering.* Apart from the magnitude of the struggle behavior, the crucial distinction between primary and secondary stuttering is that the secondary stutterer, knowing full well that he is going to have trouble with a particular word or sound, braces for the difficulty at his cords and locks them even tighter. The secondary stutterer, in other words, has anticipatory stress. He sees ahead, he scans for difficulty.

Virtually all adults are secondary stutterers. A typical stutterer will begin stuttering between two and three years of age and by the time he is five or six will have become a secondary stutterer. Stutterers from the age of seven, *when treated by a properly trained therapist,* can profitably use the techniques described in this book.

Observe that the struggling is what the child elects to do to release the locking of his cords. The stuttering is something that is learned, it is a habit. The tendency to focus tension at the vocal cords is inborn. It is an automatic reflex; stuttering is a learned or conditioned reflex. And so when researchers demonstrate that there is a tendency toward a greater incidence of stuttering in the families of stutterers than in those of nonstutterers and infer from this some form of inheritance, they are wrong. When people ask if stuttering is inherited, the answer is no. The stuttering has always been learned. What has likely been inherited is the tendency to lock the vocal cords.

This knowledge is powerful because it allows us to explain not only the inheritance findings but, for example, why approximately five times as many men stutter as women. The common mythology is that young males are subject to more stresses than young females, thus accounting for this statistic. However, studies of cultures that place early stress on females and virtually none on males still show this same ratio in regard to stuttering. The true explanation is that whenever one examines target areas, whether it be in humans or laboratory animals, one always finds differences between the sexes. We know, for example, that three times as many women focus tension at their abdominal wall muscles when under stress than do men. We also know that approximately five times as many men target stress-induced tension at their vocal cords than do women. Why these differences exist is not known as yet. One can speculate, but there are no answers. The fact that there are such differences, however, is not open to conjecture. It is directly verifiable by measurement.

Thus the odds are five times greater that one will stutter if one is a male and virtually nonexistent if one was not born with the tendency to target stress-induced tension at the vocal cords.

The vocal cords are interesting structures. They evolved a long time ago primarily as a sort of protective valve to prevent food particles from going into the lungs when one swallows. Over millions of years, they assumed another function, that of sound production. As the air comes out of the lungs, it must pass between the vocal cords, and this space is quite small. Should the space become obstructed, an individual would be deprived of oxygen, and brain damage would ensue in a few minutes. It is, therefore, very important that the vocal cords remain open, and nature recognizes this by placing many nerve endings at the vocal cords, nerve endings that detect the position, tension, and degree of openness of the cords and send this information to the brain so that it can immediately make any adjustments necessary to maintain a constant degree of openness of the cords.

Of particular interest to us are the nerve endings that detect the tension within the vocal cord muscles. When a stutterer tenses his cords to the point that they lock, this degree of tension creates a pattern of nerve impulses that flow from these nerve endings to the brain. *This pattern of nerve impulses is the trigger that fires the stuttering reflex. The object in treating stuttering is not to treat the stutter itself but rather to prevent the trigger pattern from being sent to the brain.* We cannot cut the nerve endings because this would paralyze the vocal cords. We must, however, deprive the brain of this trigger pattern, and we accomplish this by employing a set of procedures designed to subtract a great deal of tension from the cords—so much that the tension is well below the locking threshold.

The graph in Figure 2 makes this clearer. Along the horizontal axis we have units of time; on the vertical, units of vocal cord tension. The time units range from zero to four seconds and the tension units from low to high tension. Notice that at a point along the tension axis, I have indicated, by means of a horizontal line, a place I call Mr. X's threshold. Mr. X is a stutterer and this figure may be interpreted to mean that as Mr. X speaks, starting at time zero and proceeding for several seconds, should his vocal

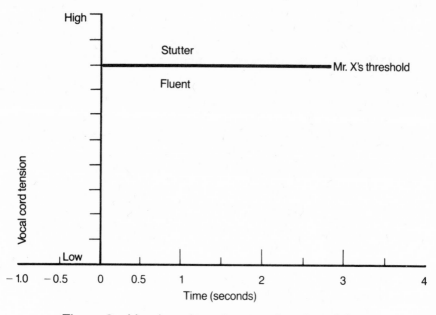

Figure 2   Vocal cord tension as a function of time

cord tension reach the horizontal threshold line, he will stutter. It is obviously very important to keep the tension below that threshold.

One of the important features of this program is that at no time do we attempt to treat stuttering. That has been tried by conventional speech therapy for decades and has proved largely unsuccessful. Stuttering is a response to a locking of the vocal cords. A good analogy is the knee-jerk response, the flying up of the foot in response to the kneecap being struck. Trying to stop stuttering by dealing directly with the stuttering makes about as much sense as trying to hold the foot down while the kneecap is being struck. The trick is to prevent the kneecap from being struck, or if it is struck, to make certain that it is struck so gently that it is below threshold.

Let us apply this figure to the analysis of a typical stuttering

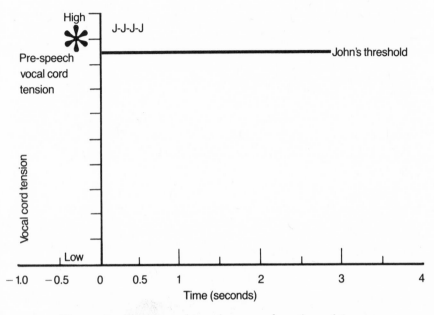

Figure 3   Vocal cord tension as a function of time

situation. At a party, a pretty young woman comes up to John Smith and says to him, "Hi. My name is Mary Jane. What's yours?" And John blurts out, "J-J-J-J-John Smith." Figure 3 shows an analysis of what has just happened. As the young woman was introducing herself, John, who in the past had found it difficult to say his first name, began to anticipate that he would have trouble once more. As a result of this anticipation, he got set by tensing his vocal cords. The question "What's yours?" was asked at −1.0— that is, before time zero. In a split second, John tensed his cords tremendously. At −0.5 the tension on his cords was so high it was above his threshold. Since his vocal cord tension was above his threshold before he spoke, it's not surprising that "J-J-J-J" came out stuttered.

How embarrassing for John. The very beginning of a relationship is marred by this sudden struggle. Is it any wonder that the socialization skills of stutterers tend to be poor and that their self-esteem in social situations is so low?

After that confrontation with Mary Jane, John decides that should another person ask him his name, he will respond, "My name is John Smith." Because, you see, he is not afraid of the words *my name is,* and he has decided that he will use them as a kind of a starter to propel him into the feared word *John.* The use of starters among stutterers is almost universal. It is a way of vibrating the vocal cords before speech begins so that they will not lock.

Winston Churchill was famous for doing this. Since he had trouble with the *e* sound in *England,* he would sustain a long *m,* or humming sound, before the *e.* Those of us who are old enough will recall his famous speech in which he said, "mmmmmEngland will never surrender." The sustained humming sound, which he did not fear, started his vocal cords vibrating and enabled him to move smoothly through the feared *e.*

The problem with starters, however, is that they don't always work, particularly if the stress is high. And frequently the stutterer starts to stutter on his starter. We occasionally see in a clinic an individual who never stutters but instead begins each sentence with an unbelievably complex string of unrelated words and sounds that are his accumulated collection of starters, starters that worked for him in the past, then failed and, instead of being discarded, were simply kept when new ones were added.

Figure 4 shows John's scheme. Remember, when the attractive female comes along (attractive females have always been high stress for him), he will, in response to the query "What's yours?" say, "My name is John Smith." Since he does not fear the words *my name is,* the tension before time zero is lower, below threshold. It is not markedly lower, however, because he knows he will eventually have to say the feared word *John.* At any rate, he begins. Notice that there is a tendency for the tension to rise with each

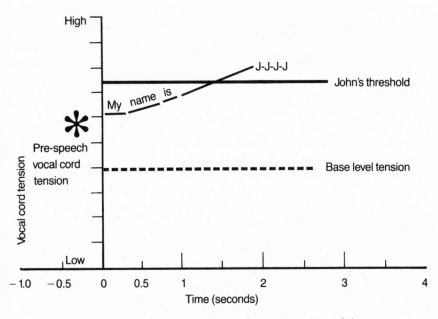

Figure 4   Vocal cord tension as a function of time

syllable in the sentence, and as he reaches the feared word *John,* there is a sudden increase in tension; he crosses the threshold and stutters.

Damn it, he thinks, sometimes it works, sometimes it doesn't. I can't predict. It fluctuates. I have good days and bad days, good hours and bad hours, good months and bad months. And this fluctuation doesn't seem to relate to anything. It seems to be out of my control.

Fluctuation is an important characteristic of stuttering. It is reported by all stutterers and is seen most vividly when the average stutterer must speak in front of an audience. Then he typically stutters severely. If he is instantly removed to an empty room, he speaks flawlessly. Retrieve him from this room, place him back in front of the audience, and the stutter returns with its former severity. In a split second, the stutterer can go from severe difficulty to none whatsoever. In this example, the situation determines the stuttering.

What happens to the stutterer when he goes in front of the audience? And what changes take place when he enters the room and is suddenly by himself? It is extremely important to understand this stuttering phenomenon. Without such understanding, any attempt at treatment is incomplete, and would probably result in failure.

Base-Level Tension on the Vocal Cords

Notice in Figure 4 a horizontal line running parallel to the time axis, reflecting the *base-level tension.* The base-level tension, an extremely important concept, is the tension on the vocal cords when a person is not speaking or planning on speaking. There are a great number of muscles within the vocal cords. Electrodes placed on these muscles would detect some degree of tension as a normal expression of being alive. However, this tension fluctuates in response to a number of factors: the time of year, the time of month, temperature, humidity, age, situation, stress at home, stress at school, stress at work, how well one has been sleeping, how well one has been eating, how well one feels—all bear upon this base-level tension. If a number of these factors are adverse at the same time, the base-level tension at that moment is high.

To speak requires further tension, called, for obvious reasons, *speech tension.* This tension is always superimposed upon the base-level tension.

If the base-level tension is high, and one speaks, thereby adding speech tension, the total tension on the cords is greater. It crosses the speaker's stuttering threshold frequently, and the speaker will likely report a difficult speaking experience.

On the other hand, if factors contributing to the base-level tension turn favorable, the tension is lowered. The addition of speech tension under these circumstances is not sufficient to reach the triggering threshold, and the stutterer therefore reports an easy speaking experience.

Thus, the good times and the bad, the fluctuation that occurs from day to day, week to week or, for that matter, hour to hour, are all due to shifting base-level tensions. When the stutterer goes in front of the audience, his base-level tension instantly increases, causing a total tension on the cords that locks them frequently, producing severe stuttering. Upon entering the empty room, he experiences an abrupt drop in base-level tension, and speech tension alone is not sufficient to reach the triggering threshold. There is no stuttering.

Now refer back to Figure 4. Imagine that a patient can be taught a technique for subtracting tension before time zero—that is, before speaking. In the next chapter, I discuss such a technique. It is known as the *air-flow technique* and was developed about a decade ago. It has been refined considerably since. It is not a technique for speech or stuttering but one that subtracts tension from the cords before the person speaks. *With the air-flow technique, the vocal cord tension can be reduced to the base-level tension.*

Figure 5 shows John Smith's proper use of the air-flow technique. Notice that the tension is now much lower as he begins his response to the question "What's yours?" The tension, as before, rises with each word, and the level of tension also accelerates with the saying of the feared word *John.* But notice that he does not reach threshold, and so he simply does not stutter. In spite of the fact that he fully expects to stutter, he suddenly finds himself unable to do so. And he wonders what went right with that feared word *John.* The answer is that nothing went right with the feared word; he tensed as much as he always did. It all went right before time zero. He simply subtracted so much tension before he spoke that as he began speaking and tensed for the feared word, that amount of tension, when added to the low level he began with,

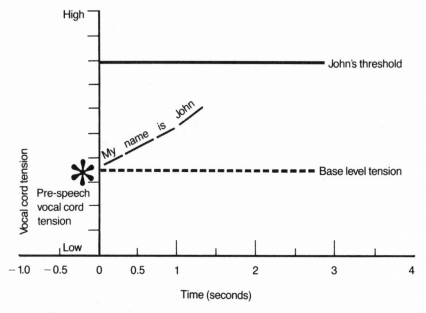

Figure 5   Vocal cord tension as a function of time

was not enough to reach threshold. And so he did not stutter.

Stutterers get set to speak by constricting their vocal cords; if they can be shown how to relax and dilate them, they can say anything.

To deal effectively with the problem of stuttering, stutterers must attack the total tension placed on the vocal cords by both of its contributing sources—i.e., the speech tension and the base-level tension. In the chapters to follow, we shall do precisely this. Chapter 2 presents a discussion of several techniques that have proven successful in the task of lowering speech tension. Taken by themselves, they are sufficient to produce fluency. But they do not give much insurance. That is, stutterers are perilously close to threshold and there is the very definite possibility that should there be a precipitous rise in base-level tension, these techniques might not subtract enough from the total tension to place stutterers below the stuttering trigger threshold.

So in Chapter 3 I present the techniques developed in the past decade that have proven effective in dealing with base-level tension. These techniques by themselves are also incapable of subtracting sufficient tension to ensure reliable fluency. Only in combination is there a sufficient reduction of tension produced within the cords to meet any stressful speaking situation.

I must, at this point, indicate that in my workshops these techniques are always modified slightly for individual differences among stutterers. In a sense, descriptions of these techniques are somewhat general since there are a number of small and subtle mistakes individual stutterers can make that can interfere with the smooth functioning of these techniques. It would be well beyond the scope of this book to enumerate these possible sources of difficulty. Such enumeration is provided in training sessions that I frequently conduct for speech therapists.

This is not a "how to" book. *It cannot replace therapy.* You need to be treated initially by a professional properly trained in these methods. The subtleties peculiar to an individual stutterer must be isolated and dealt with by suitable "fine tuning" of the technique. The professional can detect these. So I encourage any individual who stutters not to attempt to undertake the methods described herein without supervision. Without an adequate and precise evaluation of the individual stutterer, mistakes in application and execution of the techniques will undoubtedly occur. *These mistakes will lead to stuttering and cause the patient frustration.*

Most people cannot teach themselves to play classical music on the piano. They require proper instruction. Hand size, finger shape, finger dexterity, musical sense, motivation, and many other factors all bear upon this learning. So too does a host of factors prevail here. Consult Chapter 5 for information about a national organization that will put you in touch with local individuals properly trained in the administration of these techniques.

With this caution in mind, let us now begin the task of understanding the process of subtracting speech tension from the vocal cords before speech begins—the air-flow technique.

2

The Air-Flow
Technique

The vocal cords are controlled by the breathing centers of the brain. During normal, quiet respiration, they open slightly just before inhalation, then close slightly as the air flow is reversed and exhalation begins.

The opening of the vocal cords is an active process. It is the result of the contraction of a single pair of muscles located at the rear of the voice box. The exhalation phase, on the other hand, is totally passive, the inward movement of the vocal cords occurring as the muscles relax. Research has shown that the most relaxed state of the vocal cords occurs during this exhalation phase of normal, quiet respiration.

There has also been research conducted on respiration during speech. Electrodes have been placed on the vocal cord muscles to study the tension patterns associated with the production of different speech sounds. The tensions present on the vocal cords before speech have also been studied. The research reveals that the average person typically starts to tense the vocal cords between one-third and one-half second prior to the start of speech.

This fraction of a second before speech begins is most critical because it is the time during which the stutterer focuses a substantial degree of tension. If we reduce this pre-speech tension, we stand an excellent chance of keeping the total tension below the stuttering threshold.

The trick, then, is to somehow learn to exhale just before speaking, as if one were not going to speak at all but were, rather, simply engaged in yet another quiet exhalation. Somehow, what we must do is fool the brain into believing we are just taking another breath so that the brain will not develop pre-speech tension on the cords.

Flutter

Many techniques have been developed for teaching patients to produce passive air flows. Feedback devices have been developed that enable a patient to monitor the passivity of this outflow of air. The simplest, and probably most effective, is a piece of rubber tubing about a foot long. One end of the tubing is placed directly in front of the speaker's lips and the other placed in his ear. Thus the patient, as he breathes, can listen to the breath. When the air flow emerges in the totally passive manner, it produces a quality of sound in the ear that the patient learns to recognize and that is called *flutter.*

Unfortunately, each person's respiratory system is shaped differently and flutter sounds differ from patient to patient. Therefore, the patient must be trained to recognize his characteristic flutter pattern. The accomplishment of this recognition is the first phase of the air-flow technique.

Some patients can learn to produce passive air flows and acceptable flutters virtually immediately; others take substantially longer. Whatever the time involved, no further progress can be made without first attaining a consistent flutter.

Another feedback device commonly used is a tape recorder. A *special microphone* is employed for all patients, a microphone that is capable of picking up minute air flows from the mouth and recording them. The microphone is placed in front of the mouth and the air flow is tape-recorded and played back for evaluation. The patient must learn to recognize his flutter on the tape recorder.

The most important point about flutter is that it is the valid indicator of passivity. When the patient loses passivity, flutter vanishes instantly and is replaced by one of two classes of breathing sounds: pushed or squeezed flows. During workshops, pushed and squeezed flows are recorded on the patient's recorder and played back for training purposes.

Proper awareness of flutter is crucial since fluency is never a guide to the correctness of practice. For example, if a patient is practicing at home alone, his base-level tension will be much reduced and he will be fluent. Thus the patient needs some form of external objective indication of the correctness of practice. Flutter provides just such an indication.

In workshops flutter is demonstrated and each of the participants is trained in methods of producing absolutely passive outflows of air. During this extremely basic and critical phase of the program, much time is spent practicing. When flutter is produced in a consistent fashion, we move on to the next step: the production of flutter before one-syllable words. Once consistency is achieved through practice, we proceed to the production of flutter before short phrases, then before short sentences.

Slowing Down

At the start of sentences, we add an additional feature to the technique, a feature that research has shown to be as important as the passive air flow in producing tension reduction at the vocal cords. That feature is a slowing of the first syllable of every sentence.

It appears that the brain, in organizing speech, looks at the speed of the start of speech and, if it sees a quick start, tenses much the same way a sprinter tenses his leg muscles a split second before a hundred-yard dash. With a sprinter, substantial tension is required to produce a high initial acceleration of the runner's body, an acceleration crucial to success. But such acceleration is not nearly as crucial to the marathoner, and if we were to measure the tension within the runner's leg muscles a split second prior to the onset of a twenty-six-mile marathon, we would find considerably less of it.

The same holds true for the vocal cords. Quick starts require more tensing than slow starts. If our goal is to subtract as much tension as possible from the cords prior to the start of speech, then a slow start is important. In a sense, getting set to speak is the same as getting set to run a twenty-six-mile marathon rather than a hundred-yard dash.

Mastering the Technique

The combination of the passive outflow of air and the slowed first syllable produces a substantial subtraction of tension on the vocal cords before the start of speech. While the technique is simple conceptually, mastering it is not quite so easy.

In our workshops we liken the learning of this technique to the mastery of a sport. Although we are dealing with small muscles rather than large ones, the same principles appear to apply. For instance, people rarely pay attention to the way they get set to speak. Getting set, however, is important in learning most sports. Learning to get the tennis racket back into the right position is an important preliminary to being able to hit the ball squarely. Similarly, the positioning of the feet are critical to the smooth swing required in golf.

The first rule is that one must make a habit. The maneuver must be made automatic and strong. Experience has shown that it requires between sixty *thousand* and eighty *thousand* correct productions of the air-flow technique to achieve the strength of habit. This usually means a practice period of between six and eight weeks.

The patient is presented with a series of exercises to be practiced each week. Some of these involve reading selected materials. Others involve various kinds of interviews. Still others, the act of describing. All of them are designed, in one way or another, to amass the requisite number of repetitions. Such repetition is admittedly boring for the average adult. But it must be done. Mastery of the basic maneuver is crucial. The technique must become second nature.

The greatest mistake that stutterers make is to assume that because they know the technique, they can use it spontaneously and correctly whenever they need it. Such is clearly not the case. Anyone who has tried to learn a sport knows that before entering the stress of competition the basic movements of that sport must be virtually automatic. Surprisingly, stutterers, failing to equate these two learning processes, try to use the technique immediately in high-stress speaking situations and wonder why they have difficulty.

And so for two months, the patient practices the basic technique over and over, and records practice samples on a tape cassette. Each week the cassette is evaluated by a trained clinician who, based upon the evaluation, suggests a set of exercises the following week. We have discovered that all patients must be monitored by a trained clinician weekly to ensure consistency in the use of the basic technique before they proceed to progressively greater degrees of complexity in their assignments. In a sense, one must move from lesson 2 to lesson 84 without making any mistakes at each step along the way.

Toughening

One of the exercises routinely practiced is called *toughening.* It requires another person and is designed to make the stutterer resistant to the speed of the speech of those around him. There is a tendency for people to respond in kind. That is, if one is spoken to quickly, the tendency is to respond quickly. If the stutterer attempts to respond quickly, he will scarcely leave time for the implementation of his technique. Time is required to let a small bit of air flow out passively from the mouth and to slow the first syllable. Toughening teaches the stutterer to take this time.

Basically, the assistant simply asks the patient a question. The patient listens and then, employing the air-flow technique, answers it using a single sentence. In the middle of the sentence, the assistant quickly interrupts the patient to ask a second question. The patient is called upon to stop in mid-answer, use his technique again, and, employing a complete sentence, to respond, whereupon in mid-sentence he is again interrupted. This goes on for several minutes. The patient tends to speed up, discarding his technique in responding to the speedy interrupting questions thrown at him. The goal is to retain the passive air flow and to continue to slow the first syllable regardless of the speed of the questions.

I frequently tell patients at workshops that, in a sense, I wish they would all develop a peculiar form of paranoia. I wish they would believe that everyone in the world was being paid by me to toughen them. This would put them on their guard and make them highly resistant to the speed demands of the speaking world around them.

Contract

Another exercise that has proven extremely successful is called *contract*. Contract is quite simple. Once the patient is able to produce a passive air flow and slowed first syllable in short sentences, he is required to give a speech. Each sentence must be perfect, and if proper technique is not used and the speaker happens to stutter, he is required to pay the listener a dollar for every block. I tell patients that once they have the ability to abort their stuttering, it is a good idea that they pay for the privilege of inflicting upon the world around them their now unnecessary struggle behavior. Contract is to be done for three minutes at a time; one three-minute session a day for a beginner suffices.

Contract has a strong psychological impact upon the speaker. Stutterers have stuttered millions of times. It is not an earth-shattering event for them to stutter once more. But if they lose a dollar, that has great significance. Money is a primary shaper of behavior in our society, and we would be foolish not to make use of it to shape the behavior known as fluent speech.

Reapplying the Technique in Mid-sentence

As we have seen, the air-flow technique, when used at the beginning of a sentence, subtracts a great deal of tension from the vocal cords. So much so that as the person begins to speak, sees a feared word, and tenses for it, that degree of tension he develops, when added to the low level he began with, does not reach threshold, and he is fluent. This is not always the case, however. When the base-level tension is high, the air-flow technique, which can be reduced only to base-level tension, may not have subtracted enough tension, and it is possible that the person may very well stutter on that feared word in mid-sentence.

So all patients practice mid-sentence reapplications of the technique. In the workshop treatment session, patients are trained to handle difficult words by stopping, breathing in, letting some air out passively, saying the first syllable of that difficult word slowly, and then finishing the word and the rest of the sentence.

This habit of stopping to reapply the technique is of course directly the reverse of stutterers' normal tendencies. Stutterers, when confronted with a difficult word they cannot avoid, frequently speed up in an effort to rush past it rather than get caught. But this habit of increasing speed further increases the tension on the vocal cords and virtually guarantees the stutter. Stutterers do precisely the things that lead to continued stuttering!

One of the phrases commonly used in the workshop is "Practice

when you don't need it so you'll have it when you do need it."
Stutterers, when told they must practice alone, frequently respond,
"But I don't stutter when I'm alone, only with people." The response to that is: "I know that. But people are 'competition,' and
you are not up to 'competition' yet. Jack Nicklaus did not learn
to putt playing in the Master's tournament. He learned to putt
playing alone with no one watching save his coach—that is, with
no stress—until he mastered putting and then could go into high-
stress situations with the expectation that he might maintain his
technique and not be distracted."

The Concept of Hierarchy

After the six-to-eight-week period of habit formation, the patient
is introduced to the concept of the *hierarchy*. The hierarchy refers
to a way of structuring a speaking situation into versions of that
situation which are low, medium, and high along the continuum
of stress. We wish to move up the ladder of stress, experiencing
success at the lower rungs before moving on to progressively higher
ones. Using the Nicklaus analogy, we wish to move from a gallery
of five viewers to one of twenty to one of one hundred to one of
five thousand. A telephone hierarchy, for example, typically contains forty-one steps—from easiest phone calls to the most difficult.
The average stutterer, who routinely experiences a great deal of
trouble using the phone, may take a month or two to move through
the forty-one steps. When he is through, however, not only does
he have no difficulty using the phone, but he welcomes the opportunity to use it since he has lost his fear of it.

But mastery of the telephone has no implication whatsoever
for mastery of any other situation, for example, introductions. In
a sense, telephone work is like putting and introductions are like
hitting out of a sand trap. So the patient may then move on to
the introductions hierarchy, wherein he learns not only how to
introduce himself but also how to introduce one person to another.

This hierarchy may have twenty steps and may take several weeks to master.

Each situation has its own hierarchy, and the hierarchy must be developed individually for each patient by the therapist. The patient must master each hierarchy before proceeding to the next. Furthermore, the patient must not expect to do well in a situation that he has not practiced. Doing so is very much like expecting to hit out of a sand trap after having only practiced putting. One would never make that mistake in golf, but stutterers frequently make it when moving to a new speaking situation.

A typical example of this irrational thinking is seen after patients return from lunch on the first day of a workshop. Someone invariably volunteers the information "I tried the technique while ordering in the restaurant and it didn't work." My response to that observation is simply two questions: one, "Have you made a habit yet of your technique?" and two, "Have you practiced the ordering-in-the-restaurant hierarchy?" When the answer to both of these questions is no, I then ask, "What right, then, do you have to expect to do well?"

Some patients, like Dr. Carter, my co-author, are able to use the technique correctly after a very short time. We might consider them to be natural verbal athletes. The majority of patients, however, need more time to make the technique a habit and use that habit to work through their hierarchies.

Working with the patient, the therapist prevents him from having expectations of change that are out of line with reality. When one learns something new, when one forms a new habit, definite physical-chemical changes occur in the brain that are the expressions of learning. These changes develop slowly. They cannot be rushed. Patients must not frustrate themselves during this learning period since frustration serves merely to raise base-level tension and works directly against achieving goals.

Choosing the steps in the hierarchy is the responsibility of the therapist. The task of the therapist is to move the patient along as quickly as possible while preventing him from experiencing the kind of sustained frustration that would occur were the patient, left to his own resources, to make hierarchical jumps that were too great.

I tell patients in the workshop that knowing what to do and having the technique immediately available are two different things. Having the technique available means you have practiced it sufficiently. Having it available on the telephone in a high-stress speaking situation, for example, means that you've practiced it on the telephone in many situations of lesser stress.

The hierarchical method is based upon the psychotherapeutic technique known as *systematic desensitization.* This technique was developed to treat individuals who experience high anxiety or phobic reactions to certain situations. For example, it was found that a person who experiences a great anxiety about entering elevators can, if questioned by a therapist, give a subjective indication of how much fear he experiences when he imagined himself in the elevator, how much when entering one, how much when he is three steps from it, ten steps from it, and so on. The therapist encourages the patient to apply numbers to these states of anxiety, with being in the elevator given the value of 100 and being outside the building the value of 0.

The patient is encouraged to proceed up the hierarchy of anxiety by imagining himself at the lowest (no-fear) level, proceeding to the next and staying there until he reports that his fear has left him completely, then moving on to the next level and staying there until his fear is extinct, and so on.

By choosing the steps carefully and staying at each level until the fear is totally extinct, it is possible to move up the hierarchy relatively quickly and eventually extinguish the anxiety associated with that particular situation.

The interesting thing about systematic desensitization is that the results are as good when the patient merely imagines himself in a situation as they would be if he actually placed himself there.

As far as the subconscious is concerned (and all fear is ultimately stored within the subconscious), vivid imagery is perceived as reality, and a legitimate anxiety can be evoked and treated. With vivid imagery, the transfer from the unreal situation to the real world is effected automatically.

This approach has been employed successfully with all of our patients; without it, there is a great tendency to move too quickly and reach a degree of elevated base-level tension (anxiety) that prevents the patient from attending to the technique. The result inevitably is failure, frustration, and rejection of the technique.

Thus combining the air-flow technique with the principles of systematic desensitization and with a strong appreciation of the need to build habit strength has enabled a substantial majority of patients to eventually rid themselves of not only their stuttering difficulty but, equally important, their devastatingly negative psychological habit of scanning ahead for feared words, sounds, or situations.

Low-Energy Speech

No chapter on technique, however, would suffice without a description of still another technique that must be used occasionally with stutterers who demonstrate incredibly high base-level tensions at the start of therapy. These are patients who begin therapy at a level of near-panic and may not even possess enough presence of mind to attend to the technique. In these situations, I have discovered that the air-flow technique does not provide a sufficient subtraction of speech tension, and another technique becomes necessary.

You will recall that a basic theory of the air-flow technique is that it serves to subtract a great deal of tension from the vocal cords prior to the onset of speech production. Figure 6 shows a graph of a patient with an extremely high base-level tension. The distance between his base-level tension and his threshold is quite

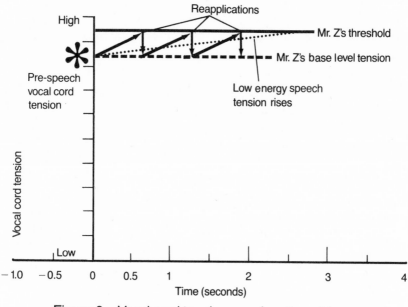

Figure 6   Vocal cord tension as a function of time

small. In other words, the arena we have to work in is meager. Recall that the air-flow technique can only bring a person's tension down to his base level. Further recall that with the start of speech the tension tends to rise with each syllable in the sentence. Figure 6 shows this situation. The diagonal lines show the individual using the air-flow technique, saying one word and then hitting the threshold. To avoid stuttering, the person would ordinarily have to stop, reapply the technique before the feared word, then go on to the next. However, the base-level tension, being so high, results in the person saying perhaps two words, then having to stop and reapply once more. The stutterer finds himself having to reapply the technique five or six times in each sentence. This proves not only tiring but aesthetically undesirable and impractical as well.

The air-flow technique only subtracts tension from the vocal cords before time zero. What is also needed is a technique for subtracting tension after time zero—that is, in the midst of speech. Techniques that subtract tension in the midst of speech distort it to greater or lesser degrees. We can, for example, use singing to produce complete fluency in any stutterer. Or, if we use whispering, we can substantially reduce or even totally eliminate stuttering in a vast number of stutterers. To produce fluency has never been a challenge. The problem is that the after-time-zero techniques heretofore available have so distorted speech that most patients reject them. I know of no stutterer who wishes to go through life singing his order in a restaurant or whispering at a party.

The object, then, is to impose a technique after time zero that produces the minimum distortion. The technique we use is called *low-energy speech.* It is defined as an extremely confidential tone of voice with reduced mouth movements. During workshops this method of speech production is demonstrated and each patient is given an opportunity to practice it. It must be practiced daily. If not, the patient forgets to use it when the stress is high, or, if he does use it, speech sounds unnatural. The key in all low-energy speech is naturalness.

Notice that low-energy speech is a backup technique, used only in extremely high-stress situations. By itself, it is totally inadequate in producing fluency, but coupled with the air-flow technique, it is powerful. If we refer to the dotted line in Figure 6, we observe that although there is still a tendency for the tension to rise with each syllable in the sentence, in low-energy speech the rise is much less abrupt and the patient can thus go further into the sentence.

Low-energy speech produces this subtraction of tension because the soft voice uses less air pressure for its production. It places less tension on the cords. The reduction of mouth movements produces a reduction in the normal spread of tension from the mouth down the neck, and this accomplishes the same thing. I call low-energy speech a safety valve, a fallback device, a guarantee of fluency. And although it is somewhat obtrusive, it is far better than singing or whispering.

I recall a patient with an extremely high base-level tension who was unable to remember to reduce his mouth movements in high-stress situations. His air-flow technique, by itself, was incapable of overcoming the elevated base-level tension. Attempts at correcting this oversight were unsuccessful and both the patient and I were frustrated.

As a final resort, I proposed an idea I had been mulling over for some time. I suggested to him that we pay a visit to an ortho-dontist colleague of mine who would put an orthodontic band on two teeth: one in the upper jaw, one in the lower. The bands would be placed at the back and would not be visible. A small wire would be attached between the two bands, a wire that could be removed at will and not employed at all during sleep and while eating, but one that could be reapplied instantaneously to hold the jaws together during speech. What I proposed to the patient were transient states wherein his jaws would be wired together as he spoke, thus preventing him from opening them wide and forc-ing the reduced mouth movements of low-energy speech.

To my surprise he agreed to this proposal. His teeth were suitably banded (two sets of bands were required, one on either side of the mouth), and he kept them in for three months, using them when he spoke. I feel that had we not been able to do this, his technique would have failed. And I am glad that he was sufficiently disgusted with his stuttering to accept this minor, though somewhat unusual, request. He eventually achieved fluent speech.

Base-Level Tension and the Need for Technique

Low-energy speech is used when the base-level tension is un-usually high; when it is average, the air-flow technique by itself suffices. When there is no stress—for example, when one is alone

Figure 7. Relation of Base-Level Tension to Speech Techniques

Stress	Speech Technique
None: Base-Level Tension = 0	None
Slight: Base-Level Tension = 25	Either slowed first syllable or passive air flow
Average: Base-Level Tension = 50	Both slowed first syllable and passive air flow
High: Base-Level Tension = 95	Slowed first syllable and passive air flow and low-energy speech

and the base-level tension is virtually zero—there is no need for technique. The amount of technique required relates to the position of the base-level tension. The higher it is, the greater the need to subtract speech tension as a countermeasure. Figure 7 shows this relationship. On the left side of the chart are different levels of stress; on the right, the amount of technique required for each of these levels. Greater technique is required for greater stress, less technique for less stress. A patient would never need the air-flow technique if he could lower his base-level tension enough so that, no matter where he spoke, it was as if he were alone.

The goal, therefore, is to use less and less technique by progressively lowering the base-level tension. The hierarchy serves to work on lowering this tension. Thus if a person no longer fears speaking on the telephone, he may discover, much to his surprise, that he no longer needs the air-flow technique on the telephone. Indeed, after a year or so of practice, most patients discover that they have been using the technique so long and so well and have gone through so many hierarchies that their base-level tension is generally greatly reduced and their need for technique is similarly reduced. They have also been using those techniques described in the next chapter to help lower base-level tension. Perhaps, too, vitamin and mineral supplements and nutritional recommendations, also discussed in Chapter 3, have further reduced their base-level tension. The result of using all these techniques is a lowering of base-level tension to the point where most patients, a year or so into the program, find that they do not stutter even though they are not using the technique most of the time. *The air-flow technique turns out not to be a permanent technique but rather a permanently available alternate mode that stutterers can go into should there be an increase in base-level tension that causes the total tension on the cords to approach the stuttering trigger threshold.*

I must caution the reader, however, that all patients at the beginning of the program and for the first six months are required to try to use the technique all the time, even though there may be some situations in which they have no trouble at all. At this stage, they need an enormous amount of practice. They must build a habit powerful enough to compete successfully against the inborn tendency to lock the vocal cords when under stress. They must have practiced the technique so long and so well and made it so much a habit that they have *earned the right* to leave it out and use it only when they need it.

If we refer back to Figure 7, we notice that for some patients it may be possible to have a base-level tension somewhere between average and none. These individuals frequently find that they cannot give up the air-flow technique altogether but can, in fact, omit a portion of it—that is, some may only slow their first syllables and others may only use passive air flows. Either of these two components by itself subtracts some tension and is often enough to keep the patient below threshold reliably.

Since virtually every stutterer, regardless of the degree of severity of the problem, is able to speak fluently when alone, we may conclude that the base-level tension and its reduction is an extremely crucial phase of any treatment program. My research now leads me to conclude that the base-level tension contributes about 70 percent to the total tension on the cords and the speech tension less than a third. If this is so, attempts to lower the base-level tension are extremely important, and the results of such lowering can add powerfully to fluency.

In the next chapter I discuss several techniques that have been shown to lower base-level tension for significant numbers of individuals. I do not attempt to outline all of the techniques since not all are needed by every individual. Instead, I highlight two of them and show how, when coupled with the simultaneous use of the air-flow technique, they can produce a powerful subtraction of base-level tension.

3

Lowering the Base-Level Tension

Stuttering: The True Social Disease

I frequently ask groups of stutterers the following question: "How many of you stutter when you speak to cockroaches? Come on, raise your hands." They chuckle and no hand goes up. "How many of you stutter when you talk to tables, chairs, cameras, fleas, paintings, bicycles?" Still no response. I then ask, "How many of you stutter when you talk on the telephone?" Most of the hands immediately shoot up. Whereupon I say, "Let me change that question a bit. How many of you would stutter on the telephone if you knew that at the other end there was a cockroach, that no person was listening, no person could listen?" And the hands drop immediately.

"This is a strange disease," I say. "People can have arthritis alone and with people, hemorrhoids alone and with people, cancer alone and with people. But people cannot have stuttering alone. Stuttering is the *true* social disease!" I continue: "How many of you started stuttering alone? And how many of you stuttered worse alone? Somehow people are the only objects in the world that have the power to raise your base-level tension to the point where you stutter. If we could turn people into cockroaches or tables or chairs, that would be the end of your difficulty. Well, I should like to show you now how to do precisely that."

I then launch into another group of questions. I create a hypothetical situation. "Suppose I came in here limping, and I had not limped yesterday. What might you say?" The answer typically offered is "What happened to you?" Or I might say, "What would you say if you suddenly saw a friend and he was wearing a cast on his arm?" And the response again might be something like "What happened to you?" Or, if you had not seen someone for a year and they had lost twenty pounds, you might make some comment about how well they looked.

I then follow with the question, "What do you say when you see someone say 'I would like a ppppppack of cigarettes'?" The typical answer is "We don't say anything." To which I may respond, "Why not, why don't you say, 'Gee fella, that's a cute stutter you've got there'?"

After the laughter, it becomes clear that people do not mention the stutterer's affliction directly to him because they are embarrassed—or more precisely, because they really do not know what to say. Instead, they act as if the person is not stuttering at all. They deny that the problem even exists. So how can you blame the stutterer for also denying that he has a problem, and for pretending that nothing is wrong? No one says anything and everyone suffers.

Several years ago I conducted an experiment with three groups of people. Group A, called "listeners," did not stutter. Electrodes were placed on their muscles and recordings were made of the tensions developed as they listened to speakers. Group B comprised fluent speakers. They entered the room individually and spoke to group A. Group C was composed of individuals who stuttered. They too spoke to group A. The same muscle recordings were made when both group B and group C spoke. The findings were predictable. Group A tensed far more when listening to stutterers than nonstutterers. Stutterers make people tense.

Part of being a stutterer is saying nothing and suffering. Stutterers and the rest of society need to talk about the problem. And those that should do the most talking are the stutterers themselves.

But virtually every stutterer is extremely hesitant to talk about his problem. The hesitation is well established at a very early age. There is an unwritten law inscribed in the mind of the child stutterer, a law carried into adulthood which states that if you talk about stuttering, something bad will happen. Opening up about stuttering is something to be feared.

Education and Demonstration

I provide all patients in the workshop with a script that I ask them to memorize. The script delineates precisely how they should explain the cause of their stuttering and how they should demonstrate their technique. This is called *education and demonstration* and it is the process by which the stutterer strips listeners of the power he has given them to tense his cords. It is the process by which stutterers turn people into cockroaches.

At refresher courses, which are conducted periodically throughout the United States, I frequently begin with the question "Who's having trouble?" Someone raises his hand. I then ask where he is having trouble. His response might be that he is having trouble at work. My next question is "Who have you educated and demonstrated at work?" The typical answer is "No one." To which I respond, "There are three things that you must do if you want to stop stuttering with people (and remember, you only stutter with people). You must educate them and demonstrate your technique to them to strip them of the power you have given them to tense your cords; you must have them toughen you so that no speed on their part can throw you; and you must make a contract with them to show that you are truly serious about wanting to get better. The most important of the three is the first."

To reinforce the importance of education and demonstration, I give examples of how the technique can transform a high-stress into a low-stress speaking situation. Here is a story I often tell: Several years ago I found myself working with three brothers who stuttered. They had decided to rid themselves of this family problem once and for all and agreed to participate in a two-day workshop at my office. During the afternoon of the first day, I received a telephone call from a local TV station. Could I appear on a show the following day at noon? They had had a last-minute cancellation. Though I had been on the show nine months earlier, and the interview had been a good one, at first I said no, I was working with patients. But then I had an idea that caused me to change my mind: I decided to appear on the show, but only if I could bring three patients with me. This was agreed to readily and plans were made to meet at the studio the following morning at 11:30.

I then informed the three brothers that they were to appear on a local TV show the following day. They would be interviewed, and probably a hundred thousand people would be watching. At first they thought I was joking, but when they discovered that I was telling the truth, their base-level tensions went through the roof. I told them not to worry, however, because I was going to arrange the interview so that they would have no difficulty.

The following morning we arrived at the studio. I spoke with the host of the program and requested that he ask me the first question and that the first question be: "Dr. Schwartz, what is stuttering?" This he agreed to do. As the program began, he asked the question, and in response I explained the cause of stuttering and demonstrated the technique for treating it in great detail. After the demonstration I engaged in a mock therapy session with the host, having him use the technique as he produced a series of sentences. He remarked how easy and simple the technique appeared to be. I agreed with him. I then demonstrated the technique with one of the brothers, pointing out to the audience present in the studio as well as at home how he breathed in, let some air out passively, and how he slowed his first syllable. The brother then generated a series of sentences as I continued to direct the viewers' attention to details of the technique. I did the same with the other brothers.

Did they stutter? Of course not! They were simply showing a technique that had been previously discussed openly. Contrast this with a program that might have begun: *This is a program on stuttering—what is your name?* (with the host pointing directly at one of the three brothers). The brother would undoubtedly have stuttered. The difference is solely the result of my having educated and demonstrated an entire audience at once.

In spite of this and other examples, I invariably sense a great resistance to educating and demonstrating, a resistance bred from years of private suffering. I tell stutterers that their resistance is real, that I understand it, and that I am sympathetic to it. But until they start to deal with stuttering openly, they will continue to be victimized by their childhood, and it will be almost impossible for them to overcome their problem.

I then distribute a button. On it is printed "I occasionally stutter, therefore I am talking slowly these days." When they first see the button, they gasp and think, I'm not going to wear that! Whereupon I say that the resistance they are experiencing is a measure of the commitment they have to hiding and suffering, and I ask them to put the button on and observe if any of them suddenly suffers a coronary.

I may then take the group to a public place—to a street corner, for example—and have them form a circle around me as I begin to speak. All of us are wearing our buttons, myself included. After a short while, passersby join the circle to listen to what I am saying. I begin to educate and demonstrate the new listeners, to show my button, and to get into a conversation with them about stuttering. I then invite the stutterers to participate in the conversation, all the while observing that everyone seems to get caught up in the spirit of the thing and become deeply engrossed in the subject matter. We then return to our workshop to discuss what happened.

The group talks about their feelings, and what they perceived the reactions of the strangers to be when shown the button and when the techniques were demonstrated to them. This activity clearly brings home one point: the fear that stutterers have about discussing stuttering is irrational and produces a chronic elevation of base-level tension. Because it is chronic, it is normal for the stutterer, and he is not aware that his base-level tension is elevated until he compares it with the euphoria he experiences when participating in the public education and demonstration.

I once treated a patient who, after the workshop, returned home, called the major newspaper in his town to request an interview with a reporter, and used the interview to educate and demonstrate. His face and button made the front page. He educated the entire city at once. He became an authority on the subject of stuttering. Stuttering became for him a subject matter and not a personal affliction. He could talk about it objectively. My co-author, Dr. Carter, was that person. He wore his button and used it to educate everyone with whom he came into contact, colleagues at the hospital where he worked, patients, orderlies, and so on. No one ridiculed him, no one lampooned him. They were all interested and supportive. And as he spoke and educated these people about stuttering, not only did his stuttering abate but so did their tensions as listeners.

I tell stutterers at the workshops that once they have a technique for stopping their stuttering, they have a moral obligation to educate people and to demonstrate their technique to them. It is not correct for the general public to harbor the notion that stutterers stutter because they are nervous or because they talk too fast, when it is clear that there are plenty of nervous, fast talkers who do not stutter, that there is something more to it, and that something is physical, a locking of the vocal cords.

Hidden stutterers—that is, stutterers who have built a life around avoiding words or avoiding difficult speaking situations— find educating and demonstrating almost unthinkable. It is the very reverse of what they have tried all their lives to avoid doing. I tell them to educate friends and family, to observe their reactions. I prepare the special script for them and have them rehearse it so they will know precisely what to say and become comfortable using the technique while following it. I remind them that people remain stutterers for a reason. They do exactly the right things to continue stuttering: they keep their base-level tension chronically elevated.

The Bathtub Technique and the Hypnosis Tape

While education and demonstration is an important technique for stripping people of the power the stutterer has given them to make him tense his vocal cords, there is still another technique of equal, if not greater, power in reducing base-level tension. It is called the *bathtub technique.* It has been used successfully with more than four thousand patients.

The bathtub technique is performed in the evening before retiring. It takes about fifteen minutes, and the fifteen minutes are considered "secure time." By "secure time" I mean that the individual will not be disturbed. He will not have to answer the telephone; someone will not come in to use the toilet. In the case of a young child, the bathtub technique is performed initially under supervision.

Three things are required: a bathtub filled with hot water, a candle in a candle holder, and a mirror. The candle is lit, placed in the holder, and put on the ledge of the tub. The mirror is placed next to it. The patient then turns out the light, enters the tub, reclines in the water so that his torso is completely submerged, breathes calmly in and out through his nose, keeps his eyes open, and stares at a spot on the wall directly in front of him. Each time the air calmly comes out of his nose, he thinks the word *one.* As he does this, he finds his mind starting to drift, starting to think other thoughts. Each time this happens, he is to bring his mind *gently* back to thinking the word "one." Since his mind is an undisciplined thing, he finds himself frequently having to bring it back to the thought. But he is to persevere for at least five minutes and steep there in the tub like a pot of tea.

The physiology behind the first phase of this technique follows: First, the knowledge that he is not going to be disturbed allows the patient to relax. Second, the hot water mechanically relaxes the muscles of his body. Third, the subdued light from the candle prevents any bright light from tensing his eyes. Fourth, fixing his eyes on a spot on the wall prevents eye-scanning movements, which is important to this exercise since eye-scanning movements have been shown to stimulate muscle tension. Fifth, thinking the word *one* over and over again will make the word meaningless. Like repeating a Hindu mantra, this prevents the patient from thinking about what he should have done yesterday and what he has to do tomorrow. Such thoughts stimulate tension.

In those five minutes, we are attempting to strip away as much muscle tension as we can, to create as much of an intra-uterine experience as we can since our mother's uterus is the safest place we ever knew: warm, moist, dark, supportive, thoughtless, relaxed. We are using an intra-uterine model as the physiological rationale for this first phase of the technique.

We now move to the second phase. The patient sits up in the tub, picks up the mirror, and positions it so that he can see his eyes. Using perfect technique, he begins to repeat the word "*relax*" slowly, using an extremely soft voice. He does this for about three minutes (usually about fifty repetitions are produced during this time).

We are now ready for the third and most important phase of the program. In it, the patient is literally going to brainwash himself. He is going to access his subconscious so that he can implant positive suggestions.

If an individual wishes to make a permanent change, he must change the self-concept of his subconscious. Stutterers have for years been telling themselves that they stutter, that they are afraid, that they cannot do many things. Their subconscious absolutely believes it. Attempting to deal with the stuttering while neglecting the subconscious virtually guarantees failure, regardless of the specific therapeutic technique employed.

A friend of mine is writing a book about dieting. It is called *Diets Work, People Don't.* Anyone who has attempted to lose weight knows that the diet itself is clearly of secondary importance. Most important are follow-through and persistence, and many factors are at work preventing these.

I learned gradually, over several years, that if I hoped to make a permanent change in stutterers, I would have to change the self-concept of the stutterers' subconscious. *The great barrier to getting information into the subconscious is the muscle tension that we carry with us like armor throughout the day.*

The first two phases of the bathtub technique are therefore designed to reduce muscle tension to a level where we can gain a clear channel into the patient's subconscious. Having done this, while still in the tub the patient reads a specially prepared series of positive statements called *affirmations.* These affirmations are prepared individually for each patient. They are read several times using the air-flow technique. Later these affirmations form the basis of a portion of a *hypnosis tape* that the patient listens to in bed before retiring and that drives these positive statements still deeper into the subconscious.

One of these affirmations is designed to provide subconscious motivation to practice. It is naïve to rely solely on the conscious desire, when the subconscious is free and accessible. Subconscious motivation is powerful but gentle. An example of this is brushing the teeth. Think of brushing the teeth as practice that we do every morning and every evening. Somehow we feel obliged to do it, as if the day would be uncomfortable or incomplete if we didn't. There is no question about our doing it. It is something that we have to do and we never call it practice. It is our subconscious at work, telling us to do it. We are almost never too tired to brush our teeth.

So too does practice become almost involuntary as the bathtub technique, coupled with the hypnosis tape, begins to affect the subconscious.

Each patient is provided with a post-hypnotic cue word that he says to himself silently just before he enters a stressful speaking situation. The cue word triggers an abrupt dropping of base-level tension to a point that begins to approximate the degree of tension the person experiences in the bathtub. Many stutterers, when saying this cue word, experience a profound drop in base-level tension, to the point where they appear to themselves to be alone, in spite of the fact that they may be making a presentation before a group. Their fluency is then guaranteed.

The Importance of the Subconscious

The importance of the subconscious must not be minimized. Sometimes the subconscious mind can be totally at odds with the conscious mind. I recall treating a young man from San Francisco. He was a financial genius and had been promoted repeatedly, until, at the age of thirty-three, he was earning a substantial income. In addition, he was an entertainer. His hobby was mime, and he gave frequent performances for children at local hospitals. He also stuttered severely.

This young man participated in one of my workshops, learned the technique easily, and immediately set to work practicing to develop habit strength. He complied in all respects with the prescribed practice regimen.

However, he made no progress. I was mystified. All patients who practice show progress, and show it immediately. Had he been mentally retarded or had cerebral palsy I would have had an explanation. But here was an extremely intelligent and motivated young adult doing exactly what he was supposed to do and still showing not one jot of improvement.

I saw him several months after the start of treatment at one of our regularly scheduled refresher courses. His wife accompanied him (we invite spouses to attend the workshops as well as the refresher courses). He had been married for six years, and the marriage apparently had not been a good one for her. I observed that she continuously berated him. Nothing he did was good enough for her. She bickered and complained about everything: the way he stood, how he dressed and combed his hair; even his choice of words seemed to require her constant derisive attention.

He, on the other hand, was deeply in love and considered himself the luckiest man alive to be married to such a "wonderful" woman. After all, was he not a severe stutterer and hadn't she been the only person who seemed not to be bothered by it and to see the "true" person underneath it all?

More months passed. Still no progress. He began to have serious doubts about ever getting better. He became depressed. I saw him at the next Bay Area refresher course. She was with him, and in her verbal abuse was as abrasive and unrelenting as ever. But still he appeared to take it with an equanimity based upon a limitless love he still professed for her.

Later I was told by one of his fellow patients that a month after the refresher course his wife had come to him and revealed that she had been seeing another man for more than a year and that she planned to leave with him that very day.

My patient was stunned, shocked, devastated, demoralized . . . *and he never stuttered again!*

While his conscious mind had been filled with denial, his subconscious mind had perceived all along what was happening. His wife's constant harassment served to continuously drive his base-level tension up, and her sudden departure produced an abrupt and considerable drop in its magnitude. The result was an immediate fluency for a profoundly unhappy man!

Yet another example of the independence of the conscious and subconscious minds can be found in a description of the way I stopped smoking. It happened about a decade ago. Prior to that I had been a heavy smoker—cigarettes, cigars, pipes—for about seventeen years. I was hooked.

Several weeks prior to stopping, I had made the acquaintance of a research psychologist who was employed, as I was, at New York University Medical Center. He had been conducting research with a population of emphysematous patients, individuals who had lost a substantial amount of lung tissue, typically as a result of a life history of heavy smoking.

As we walked through the emphysema ward I was impressed by the patients' struggles to stay alive. Oxygen was available everywhere, and these unfortunate souls found that the merest exertion would send them scurrying for it. The sight was frightening and I was deeply affected.

The psychologist showed me post-mortem photographs of lung tissue, tissue that looked like bubbling black asphalt on a hot summer day. I could not believe that that shiny, black gelatinous mass I saw in the photographs had once been pink and firm.

Then I saw an individual whom I shall not forget. A man in his late fifties, he had suffered the removal of his voice box as the result of cancer. He could no longer speak and was required to breathe through a small hole in the front of his neck, a hole that passed directly into his windpipe. He wrote instead of speaking.

As I walked by, he tapped my arm and wrote something on his pad: "Got a cigarette?" I reached into my shirt pocket and offered him one. He removed the oxygen tube, which had been in the hole in his neck, inserted the cigarette in its place, lit it, and took a deep breath. With one hand on the cigarette and one on the pencil he wrote, "Thanks, they don't allow smoking here, but what the hell."

The next day I stopped smoking. Did I want to stop? No. Had I consciously planned to? No. My subconscious had made the decision for me. And, as a result, in the ensuing decade, I have never once had the desire to smoke. Oh yes, you can stop smoking as a result of a conscious decision, but the difference is that you always have to fight the desire to start again. If the subconscious has not made the decision, the attraction is always there.

Thus the subconscious always plays a crucial role in the production and maintenance of permanent change. During the first several years of treating stutterers, this conclusion was driven home to me repeatedly. I would teach a patient the air-flow technique and produce an immediate fluency. If the patient's stuttering had been severe, the change would constitute a particularly marked contrast to his former speech. It would be both dramatic and abrupt, and the patient and his friends and family would be much impressed.

But the subconscious would not. The subconscious appears to make no value judgments. Stuttering is not good or bad, it's simply what is. And when the patient abruptly ceased stuttering, the subconscious would become "concerned." The self-concept of the subconscious had been violated, and the violation constituted a threat to the well-being of the individual.

When such a threat occurred, the subconscious would have recourse to just one defense: it would raise the base-level tension. The patient would experience a marked increase in his state of anxiety.

He would then call, saying that he had awakened that morning to find himself experiencing great anxiety. He did not know the source of the anxiety but felt it was somehow related to his sudden fluency. It is well known in learning psychology that *all newly learned behaviors are lost under conditions of stress.* The elevated state of anxiety was an attempt on the part of the subconscious to restore its self-concept as a stutterer by causing the patient to give up his newly learned behaviors. I saw this occur repeatedly. Former severe stutterers, now completely fluent, would call me on the special hotline number I had given them. They had been using the technique from one to eight months, were pleased with the results, and had expected that they were well on the way to becoming permanently fluent.

Now, suddenly, here was this strange anxiety, almost terror. Many of them felt that if they started stuttering again, their anxiety would decrease, and for about 6 percent of the patients this is precisely what happened. I called it the "assault of the subconscious," and I have recognized it as one of the two major sources of relapse (a discussion of the second source follows).

To combat it, a professional hypnotherapist is employed to prepare a tape that addresses the patient's subconscious directly. The tape is used at night, and its primary purpose is to convince the subconscious that the technique is good, that it should be welcomed, and that its continued use provides more and more pleasure for the individual. The tape, to be listened to nightly for several months, is reported to have had a cumulative effect. Since its employment, the occurrence of the "assault of the subconscious" has dropped to almost zero, with a commensurate increase in long-term success rates.

Fluency Without Practice: A Common Cause for Relapses

A lowered base-level tension, produced by an excellent air-flow technique coupled with both education and demonstration and the bathtub technique, produces a high degree of fluency in patients and can set the stage for the second classic form of relapse. Unlike the type just described, wherein the patient relapses as a result of anxiety produced by the subconscious, in this instance the relapse is caused by sloppy technique engendered by a total *absence* of stress. Here is an example: The patient masters the techniques for lowering speech tension and base-level tension. After four months he is completely fluent in every situation. He thinks he is cured and stops practicing. He ceases attending club meetings, he stops sending tapes. He simply quits. In all respects, he has given up the very activities that produced his fluency in the first place.

A month goes by. His technique is excellent, his base-level tension is low, and he is completely fluent. Another month passes. Now his speech technique is beginning to drift a bit. The air flow is losing some of its passivity. He is inconsistent in slowing his first syllable. But he hasn't stuttered at all because his base-level tension is low.

Another month passes. Now his technique has drifted considerably, his air flows are clearly not passive, and he almost never slows his first syllables. But he still does not stutter because he continues to "ride" on his lowered base-level tension.

The important point is that since he hasn't stuttered, he thinks that his technique is still good; what he clearly does not know is that it ceased being good two months earlier. He is being fooled by his fluency.

One day he suddenly finds himself in a multiple stress situation. His base-level tension goes up. Someone asks him a question quickly, he turns quickly to respond, and he stutters. No problem, he thinks. I'll just use my technique. And he stutters again. He tries the technique a second time and stutters a second time. When this happens, he suddenly thinks that his technique has just stopped working, and when this realization occurs—at that very instant—he loses all confidence in it and his base-level tension shoots upward instantly. He stutters worse than he has in years. And because he disengaged himself from fellow patients and his therapist several months earlier, he is too embarrassed to return to them stuttering as badly as he does, and he slinks away as some miserable hulk of a relapse, in violation of the eleventh commandment, which states: Thou shalt not be conned by fluency!

Lowering Base-Level Tension with Vitamins and Minerals

The base-level tension can also be lowered through the effect of certain vitamins and minerals. Some research shows that vitamins C and B-complex and the minerals calcium and magnesium are capable of lowering muscle tensions for *some* people. It is important to stress that these substances do not affect all individuals, and therefore an experiment is required to determine whether or not they benefit a particular individual.

The amount to be taken is extremely important and depends upon a number of factors: age of the patient, bone structure, body weight, body type, subjective impression of stress, and an impression of the severity of the stutter. I strongly caution the reader against indiscriminate use of these substances, for although no known toxicities have resulted from the amounts generally recommended, such experimentation is best done carefully and with the support of one's physician, especially if the individual is taking medication.

When the appropriate dosage of both the vitamins and minerals is determined, the patient takes these substances for six weeks, after which the amount is reduced by half. A resulting deterioration in speech performance is viewed as a sign that the vitamin-mineral combination is of value to that individual. If there is no perceived degradation in speech performance after one week of 50 percent reduction, the dosage is further reduced to the point of total elimination. Again the speech performance is assessed for degradation.

Only one in four patients shows a positive effect from the vitamin and mineral regimen. Within that group, some show slight effects (which are probably largely placebo effects) while others show substantial ones. Indeed, for a very small number of patients, the administration of the vitamin and mineral program lowers their base-level tension enough to bring them below their threshold, and they become fluent. For these people, life becomes simple.

But I must again point out that the number of patients who benefit to this extent is extremely small, while a fairly constant one-quarter of the patients have shown some improvement.

Food as an Elevator of Base-Level Tension

The final subject generally discussed at the workshop is the role of food as an elevator of base-level tension. We are all familiar with the fact that some individuals show strong allergic reactions to certain foods. An individual allergic to shellfish may experience dizziness, profuse sweating, flushing, disorientation—a variety of somatic responses.

What we may not be familiar with, however, is the fact that a large number of individuals may show subtle allergic reactions to certain foods, reactions so small that they typically take place beneath conscious awareness. They are known as *microallergic reactions,* and the substances that produce them are called *provocative foods.* Let me give an example. If I get up in the morning and take my pulse, on the average it is 72. If I then take a small piece of hard-boiled egg, put it in my mouth, chew it thoroughly for thirty seconds, swallow, and immediately take my pulse again, it is no longer 72 but is now 86. My pulse rate has gone up fourteen beats per minute because my body perceives hard-boiled eggs as a mild toxin and my pulse rate increases as my body's attempt at detoxification takes place.

This dramatic increase in pulse rate is of interest to us because there is a strong correlation between the increase in pulse rate associated with the eating of certain foods and an increase in muscle tension. If I were to place electrodes on the muscles of my body, I would observe an increase of tension shortly after placing the hard-boiled egg in my mouth. If I ate hard-boiled eggs frequently, I would be experiencing a nutritionally based chronic elevation of base-level tension.

It is a simple matter to test for provocative foods. It can be done at home, and each person must make the test for himself since provocative foods vary from person to person and no generalizations can be made. Here is the test: Take your pulse by counting the number of beats per minute. Place a food in your mouth, chew it vigorously for thirty seconds, then swallow. Immediately take your pulse again. If your pulse rate has gone up more than eight beats per minute, the food is considered to be provocative and you are advised to remove it from your diet.

You can test one food every three hours or one food at each meal. It should, of course, be the first food at that meal. Since there are not so many different foods that you eat all the time, it is possible to assay your diet in about two weeks. This is an important test that should be done by everyone. Even nonstutterers report that if they routinely eat several provocative foods and then eliminate them from their diet, they experience a marked increase in their sense of well-being. When just one provocative food is added to the diet of laboratory animals, on the average they do not live as long as animals given an identical diet except for the offending food.

Begin your determination of provocative foods by examining coffee and tea. In these instances, the liquid is swizzled around in the mouth for thirty seconds before being swallowed. Caffeine is frequently a culprit.

About one in five patients shows at least one provocative food. A small number of patients who eliminated their provocative foods found themselves below threshold without having to use any other technique. Again, for these individuals, life becomes simple. While this number may be quite small, the number of people reporting at least one provocative food is not. So all patients are encouraged to look for and attempt to root out all provocative foods from their diets.

Base-level tension is the source of more than two-thirds of the total tension placed on the vocal cords. The techniques described in this chapter—education and demonstration, bathtub, vitamins and minerals, and food-testing—constitute the major tools employed in the assault on base-level tension. In the next chapter, we shift our attention to an extremely important group of factors necessary to making a permanent change—the external support system. Without it, the patient is left to fend for himself. This is dangerous since very few patients possess sufficient power within themselves to effect permanent changes alone; they need the external support system.

4

The External
Support System

I have already mentioned that stutterers rarely, if ever, stutter alone. In view of that, any attempt to make a permanent change in stutterers that disregards the importance of the outside world—that is, the world of speaking individuals—is destined to fail. The outside world must be employed in a constructive manner to assist the stutterer in overcoming his problem. To that end, considerable effort has been expended in the establishment of a system of interrelated supports. The system has been refined and expanded over the past decade and is now viewed as an integral component of the overall rehabilitation program.

There are two forms of external support. The first is professional; the second is self-help.

Professional Support: Therapists, Refresher Courses, and the Stutterer's Hotline

The professional support system is made up of three components. The first of these is the therapist, whose job it is to monitor the patient's performance weekly and to guide the patient through each speaking-situation hierarchy. This professional is a specially trained individual with several years of clinical experience working with stutterers. After a period of several months of special training, the therapist becomes expert at detecting *all* of the subtle variations in flutter that patients can exhibit as well as the many details required to move quickly past basic training and on through the situation hierarchies.

It is the job of the therapist to give the patient a new assignment each week. Segments of the assignment are then recorded on a tape cassette and sent to the therapist for evaluation. The evaluation is recorded on the patient's cassette, together with the next week's assignment, and the tape is returned. This exchange process between therapist and patient lasts from eighteen to twenty-four months.

It must be emphasized that it does not take a year and a half to two years to stop stuttering; that goal can be achieved in several months. What does take the time is the extinction of the habit of scanning ahead for feared sounds, words, or speaking situations. The "scanner" must go to sleep, and since bad memories die slowly, the stutterer must be patient. In the course of working with thousands of stutterers, I have learned that if a patient stops practicing when he no longer stutters, but still scans, he relapses.

Stuttering is a mechanical event that occurs in response to the attainment of a threshold level of tension on the vocal cords. The air-flow technique is a mechanical technique that subtracts tension from the vocal cords to a point below threshold. Such mechanical techniques can only be learned with practice. The more practice the individual puts in, the more quickly he attains mastery of the mechanics of the technique, and the more quickly he becomes fluent. Attaining total extinction of anticipatory stress, on the other hand, is a psychological event, which apparently cannot be rushed, and which usually takes between eighteen and twenty-four months to accomplish.

One example may suffice. Several years ago a young man with a relatively severe stutter dropped out of college because he was unable to participate in class speaking situations. His stuttering also seriously affected his ability to socialize. He felt himself, and was, an outsider.

He attended one of my workshops and appeared eager to master the technique so that he could return to the university in time for the start of the following semester. He performed well throughout the two-day session and afterward came to me with a rather unusual request. Instead of practicing for about an hour a day, as is the custom with patients, he wished to practice eight, ten, or even twelve hours each day. He lived at home and fortunately did not have to work, so he had the time to devote to practice.

I prepared a special set of assignments for him that I called minimarathons. He would practice for thirty minutes, then stop for thirty minutes, all day long. In other words, fully half of each day would be devoted to practice. He agreed to this schedule. His target date for reentry was a mere three months away, and he wished to return with a reasonable degree of control over his speech.

He approached his practice assiduously, and this relatively severe stutterer became totally fluent in every speaking situation in eleven weeks. He continued to practice until he achieved total extinction of all scanning behavior; this took a full twenty months. The interesting point is that although he was able to mechanically stop stuttering relatively quickly, he was intelligent enough to understand that had he stopped practicing with the attainment of fluency—that is, after eleven weeks—he would surely have relapsed. The full conversion of his subconscious, the extinction of all anticipatory stress, took close to two years! Such is the disparity between the mechanical and psychological components of this technique.

The second form of professional assistance is the refresher course, conducted periodically throughout the United States. All patients benefit from this face-to-face contact with their therapist. Many of them report that personal contact with a therapist every few months does much to remotivate them to continue practicing.

At these refresher courses, each patient stands and gives a short speech, after which his technique is critiqued. The critique often involves a detailed analysis of subtle aspects of facial expression as well as of body movement associated with use of the technique. Since these visual components cannot be readily detected by the therapist when listening to the tape cassettes, these face-to-face meetings are essential.

In addition, the refresher course allows time for dealing in depth with particular questions raised by the patients. Further, it provides an opportunity for discussing highly refined strategies for handling unusual and high-stress speaking situations. For example, one patient worked in a nuclear electric generating plant. He was an evening supervisor and virtually ran the plant. His stuttering was controlled, but his greatest fear was that in the event of a crisis, when called upon to give a long and complex series of commands rapidly, he would find himself unable to do so. While he hoped that such a crisis would not occur, he lived in fear that, if it did, it would prove devastating not only to him but to those who relied on him. This knowledge weighed heavily upon him, and he thought a great deal about changing jobs.

I suggested that he stage simulated emergencies or full-blown dress rehearsals, and that he conduct these often to get practice speaking under such circumstances. Such rehearsal was, of course, a routine procedure at the nuclear installation. What he did was to increase the frequency of such staged emergencies. His goal was to make them as vivid as possible, to attempt to experience the full set of emotional responses that might occur in such a situation.

Six months later I received a letter from him informing me that a true emergency had occurred and that as a result of the practice, he had handled it flawlessly. He was proud of his accomplishment. It had not gone unnoticed, and he had been promoted to a new position, one that required no such need to speak under stress. His practice had moved him into a low-stress speaking situation.

The third and, by far, most important application of professional assistance is the unique support provided by a special hotline number established for stutterers employing the air-flow technique (the number is given on page 83). At any time—day, night, or weekend—a stutterer knows that he can call a special toll-free number and receive assistance with any problem related to his speech. This hotline has proved to be a boon to many patients who use the air-flow technique. Stutterers can call about a particular assignment, or if they are having a bad day, or when they are worried about an upcoming speaking situation and wish a strategy for maximizing their success.

For example, several years ago I treated a patient who worked for the State Department. He had done quite well in his career because he was largely a closet stutterer. But his career was severely hampered because he was unable to learn a second language, which is a requirement for advancement in the State Department. The difficulty was that in the learning of the second language he would not have the facility to word-substitute. He would have to say all of the feared sounds, and his anxiety over this prospect had grown to gargantuan proportions; the mere thought of having to study a foreign language was terrifying.

He wanted to learn French, but all attempts in the past had failed miserably. Now he had been practicing the air-flow technique for six months and felt he was ready. In the State Department one can learn a foreign language intensively—that is, one can practice, usually in class but sometimes one-on-one with a teacher for six hours a day for a number of weeks until mastery of the basic elements of conversation in that language is achieved. The first day of his training began. The session went well for the first half-hour, and then he hit his first serious block. His base-level tension shot up and he found himself suddenly unable to continue. All of his old fears about learning a second language returned with their full ferocity.

He asked to be excused, went to the nearest pay phone, and

dialed the toll-free hotline number. A therapist responded and provided him with the following instructions. He was to return to his instructor and immediately educate and demonstrate. He was to use low-energy speech throughout the language sessions. He was to call the hotline as often as necessary. On the first day he called several times. On the second, he called twice. He successfully completed the course.

We have discovered that these three forms of professional external support are crucial to the establishment of a permanent change. Far too often, in other therapy programs, the patient is left to fend for himself once the attainment of fluency is achieved. I, on the other hand, view such attainment as merely the first step in the program. It is naïve to suppose that an individual who has stuttered for twenty years can make a permanent change in a few weeks or months. The attainment of permanency is signalled by the extinction of all anticipatory stress, and such extinction takes years to achieve. The weekly monitoring of tapes by a trained professional is a must; the refresher courses are vital; and the hotline, more often than not, has been the crucial component in determining success or failure for a patient. All of these forms of support are necessary, and all of these, fortunately, are now available to stutterers in the United States.

Nonprofessional Support: Clubs, Monitors, and Banquets

While professionals are of inestimable value in the external support system for stutterers, nonprofessionals are just as important. There are three ways stutterers can get support, motivation, and help from nonprofessionals.

First, *clubs* for air-flow users have been established in most major cities in the United States. Most of the clubs meet twice a month and act as powerful support groups. The meetings are held at local hospitals, churches, or libraries in rooms set aside for the purpose.

A strict meeting format is followed. The purpose of the format is to provide the maximum opportunity for everyone to speak and the maximum motivation to continue the regimen of daily practice. A rotating leadership system prevails, allowing each club member to lead a meeting. Various exercises are performed. Inspirational speeches are given. A variety of simulated situations are created, and members have the opportunity to practice within them. At the meetings, members break up into subgroups and work on various aspects of their technique. Throughout the meeting, technique is critiqued and all members are encouraged to do their very best.

After a short while the club meeting itself ceases to be very stressful for the members. At this point advanced members begin to function as a sort of miniature lecture bureau. For example, in each club a nucleus of advanced members arranges to give a group lecture on stuttering to various organizations. They may lecture at a variety of fraternal organizations, a speech-therapy class at a local college, or a women's group. Their goal is not only to educate and demonstrate a public that needs such knowledge, but, in the process, to use the support of the club as a tool by which they broaden their public-speaking ability and gain self-esteem. Newer members in the club aspire to join these minilecture bureaus and, once they have become sufficiently expert in the use of the technique, are welcomed into the bureau.

Many club members have also given interviews to local newspapers and have spoken on radio and television as well. To go from being a person who stutters to one who receives applause as a result of a public lecture represents the most extensive change in self-concept that can be achieved. The individual who accomplishes this goal has gone so far psychologically that the possibility of relapse is extremely remote.

Many of the participants in the air-flow club meetings go on to join a national public-speaking organization called Toastmasters. Here they have an opportunity to give a speech before an audience every week. A number of air-flowers have become presidents of their local Toastmasters chapters, and others have won regional public-speaking competitions.

One patient in particular is noteworthy. This fifty-seven-year-old woman attended a workshop in Lake Tahoe. She had been a violent stutterer, so violent that for years she had been required to wear a neck brace each day, since the ferocious backward thrusts of her head as she stuttered were destroying her cervical spine.

She learned the technique at the workshop and returned to her home in Whitehorse, in the Yukon Territory, where she educated and demonstrated everyone. She wore her button and religiously practiced the tension techniques until she became totally fluent.

Four months after attending the workshop she joined a local Toastmasters. Several months later she entered and won a local public-speaking competition. A year after that she came in second for all Canada.

Later I conducted a workshop in Whitehorse. The woman had become quite a celebrity in the territory and was running for political office. Her husband was Area Superintendent for Federal Parks. One afternoon I found myself seated at the front of a small helicopter, touring the wilderness and looking for grizzlies as we skimmed at treetop level over a mountain range. I thought that if I was ever going to start stuttering, it would be now. After we had landed at a campsite high in the mountains, her husband told me that the three greatest moments in his life were when he married his wife, when their first child was born, and when she returned from that workshop in Lake Tahoe.

While clubs are invaluable for patients wishing to recover from stuttering, a form of local or daily external support is also needed. The environment around the stutterer must be shaped to provide assistance. To that end, I have established what is known as the *monitor system*. A monitor is a person—be it a spouse, parent, or friend—who has a vital interest in the stutterer. A monitor knows the details of the treatment program. He or she has read the training manual provided for each patient and understands all of the features of the treatment.

A monitor has a sort of mental checklist. The monitor asks the patient whether he has been toughened that day, for example; if he hasn't, the monitor toughens him. The monitor may ask to hear what the therapist has said on the last cassette. The monitor may practice with the patient and be with him as he uses the technique in a department store or goes through the telephone hierarchy. The monitor is to be considered a kind of surrogate parent, a mother or father who is intimately involved with the child's homework. We have discovered that patients make much greater progress if there is someone at home and/or at work or school who is intimately involved with the rehabilitation program. People have a lot more power to change when they are with another person rather than alone. As Ma Barker said when she was teaching her sons how to rob banks, "Remember this: when you rob a bank, one man can cover one person, but two can cover twenty!"

The same is true for the stutterer. Somehow he has much more power when he feels he is not alone, when someone is with him to encourage and support him continuously.

From time to time a stutterer reports that he lives alone, that he knows virtually no one, that his work is done in isolation, and that he cannot think of who might be a suitable monitor. I suggest that he go out and buy one, that he pay a high-school student a few dollars an hour to function as a monitor. At all costs, he must not try to succeed alone. He is to think of the stutterer inside himself as a sort of child subpersonality, one that needs parenting.

We have repeatedly discovered that monitors are *crucial* to the establishment of success and that patients who attempt to succeed alone court disaster. Although it is possible for some individuals to succeed by themselves, their number is small. The general suggestion is: get a monitor. And if you can find two, you are twice blessed.

Each year, throughout the United States, *banquets* are held in a number of cities. They celebrate the achievements made by students of air flow. After dinner, thirty individuals present short speeches on a topic related to the theme "How My Life Has Changed." These speeches illustrate how far these individuals have come in changing their lives. A call for speakers for an upcoming banquet is usually announced a month in advance; the first thirty to respond are chosen. In recent years, far more have responded than time was available for. Those who are "shut out" one year are given top priority for the following year's presentation. I recall one patient who felt so disappointed at not being able to speak at a Washington, D.C., banquet that he submitted his name for one in New York, was accepted, and flew up for the dinner.

Individuals who have shown an interest in learning air flow but who have not yet done so are invited to attend a banquet and listen to the speakers after the dinner. Many of these stutterers are skeptical about being able to recover. They have had many therapies in the past, and none of them has ever worked or, if they did work, did so only for a short time. As these individuals hear one success after another, a glimmer of hope begins to develop within them. Later, they seek treatment.

What follows are transcriptions of three typical speeches collected from recent banquets. The first is the story of a police officer:

———

Actually I remember myself always stuttering. Impressions would stick out in my mind of times I had stuttered. These would always be embarrassing to me. Most of my friends didn't really think I stuttered at all, because, I guess, of the way I would substitute words. But only I knew how many times I kept quiet because of the fear of stuttering.

At about nineteen, after I graduated from high school, stuttering really started to bother me, and I knew I had to seek some kind of help. I just didn't want to stutter anymore. So I began seeing a speech therapist, who provided some help. We discussed certain tricks I could use, the different kinds of stutterers, when stuttering would occur, etc. Everything but a cure, because there wasn't any. This therapy continued for approximately three years with some success. Maybe not success in decreasing my stuttering, but in accepting it and feeling better about myself, even though I still stuttered.

At age twenty I took an examination for patrolman. I had scored well on the written, and on the physical I scored over 90 percent. As in all police examinations, a psychological test is required. This meant an oral interview with the police psychiatrist. I remembered going into that office expecting the worst—that I would stutter. Well, needless to say, I did stutter. At the end of these interviews the psychiatrist either writes a good report on the applicant or rejects him. The following is a quote from the doctor's report:

"He has a problem with stammering and stuttering which becomes extremely intense during the interview. He is not in touch with his emotions. It is my impression that in periods of stress he would have a tendency to use poor judgment."

Needless to say, I was disappointed in this rejection, but more, I felt angry. I felt that stuttering was the cause again.

About a year later, after a court hearing and visits with other psychiatrists, I was offered the job of patrolman, which I accepted, still stuttering. Evidently they rejected the first doctor's report as unsubstantial.

There were times on the job where I couldn't talk into the walkie-talkie. I dreaded the thought of having to go to court. My fellow patrolmen were starting to notice, which bothered me. Most would offer suggestions and tried to be helpful, but it was slowly taking its toll. After I had been on the job about two and a half years, during which time I had thought about quitting the police force many times, my father saw an article in the *New York Daily News* advertising a book called *Stuttering Solved*, by Dr. Martin Schwartz. I went out the next day and bought the book. I had honestly thought that this was my last chance, my last hope. Anyway, to make a long story short, I read the book, called Dr.

Schwartz, and made an appointment, at which time I was scheduled to come back in a few months and start the "treatment" or
program.

After the first day with Dr. Schwartz, I knew that this was
it. There was a way. I was told, and I believed, that just because
you stutter doesn't mean that there is something mentally wrong
with you. Knowing that was very important to me. Dr. Schwartz
stated that stuttering was a habit, not a mental disorder.

Anyway, on the second day with Dr. Schwartz, I taped a
television talk show for WNYC, channel 31. I can remember sitting
down and the cameraman saying, "Five seconds till showtime."
I thought my heart was going to come out of my chest, I was so
damn nervous. When it was my turn to speak, I just sat back and
used the technique, and it was instant fluency. I had surprised
myself. I remember after that show was over, being so proud of
myself and really feeling as though I could do anything.

Since that show about a year ago, I have been in court
several times, I have worked in the radio room dispatching radio
cars around the city, and even read a passage from the Bible in
church at a friend's wedding, in front of a large congregation.

In the past, these experiences would have brought on tre-
mendous feelings of terror and anxiety. Now I actually look forward to such situations.

I have treated several policemen over the years and, as a group,
they have done beautifully. The need for perfect speech in extremely high stress situations is an important factor behind their
determination.

The second individual is older, a thirty-five-year-old computer
professional, and had been stuttering for a bit longer. His story
contains many of the features common to the life history of the
stutterer. Here we have a biography of the typical stutterer to
whom stuttering was a lifelong pattern. In a sense, this is the ar-
chetypal story:

I remember a childhood friend asking me why I talked funny sometimes. The question surprised me, but it was the beginning of an awareness that I did have difficulty speaking at times. This was at the age of eight. I soon realized that I was having difficulty in school particularly, and was enrolled in speech therapy for the first time in the second grade. I met other children with the same problem at the institute. I attended therapy sessions for over a year, but I'm not sure what effect it had.

By the third grade I had begun to experience real humiliation and frustration in classroom reading situations. Reading and speaking before a group became an experience to be feared. I was aware of laughter as I stuttered my way through repetitious sentences. Words on a page would blur before my eyes and lose their meaning. The harder I tried, the more my fluency disintegrated. The next few years were the worst. I considered pretending to be a mute as a way of avoiding the uncontrollable stuttering which was causing me embarrassment and shame. I had heard someone say that I would outgrow it eventually, and this was the hope I held on to.

I remember a period of several months when speech without stuttering was impossible. I clung to a few short answers which I felt safe in saying: "Same here," "I don't know" were a couple.

I began to substitute words and phrases for those I knew would cause me trouble, and gradually built up a fairly successful ability for scanning and switching to improve fluency. Of course, there were still unavoidable situations in which I could not substitute, and the blockages were interminable at times. An article I had to read to the class as a freshman in high school is still fresh in my mind. It had dealt with abbreviations and acronyms used for agencies and companies. It took me great lengths of time to stutter through the letters, which appeared over and over again. I managed to get through part of the first page before the laughter was apparent. I would have laughed myself if I hadn't felt so miserable. I finally looked at the teacher in such a pleading way that he had someone else finish reading for me.

At home, things were little better. I dreaded the use of the phone. It was something I used only under duress. To be home alone and hear the phone ring was traumatic. Each time I faced a decision to just let it ring or force myself to pick up the receiver. Inevitably, when I did answer it, my stuttering was disastrous.

As a teen-ager, I still felt I would outgrow my affliction. I couldn't imagine being a stuttering adult. As a sophomore in high school I decided to return to the institute for therapy. After several months of group therapy I still didn't understand what we were doing, what we were trying to do, or whether I was improving. I stopped going.

I chose a technical area of study in college, since it was clear to me and my counselors that I would function best where oral communication would not be a burden. I periodically reviewed the literature on speech therapy for hints and theories relating to my problem. I realized that I was not going to outgrow it after all, and tried to plan accordingly.

As an adult, my pattern was still to avoid people and situations which gave me trouble. I was quite fluent at times. The phone remained an obstacle. Extreme nausea, rapid heartbeat, sweating and shortness of breath were some of my reactions to simple phone calls. Clever substitutions and various distractions (for example, writing words on a chalkboard) got me through many situations. Some friends of mine were unaware that I had a problem. They could never guess the energy and planning I put in to keep my speech "under control."

About a year ago, my parents sent me a clipping on the air-flow technique and Dr. Schwartz. I was curious enough to read the book. It became an exciting experience as I saw my frustrations catalogued and explained in those pages. Understanding the problem was almost satisfaction enough; I was hesitant at first to commit myself to the possibility of undergoing therapy. I finally resolved that if I were ever to try to beat stuttering again, this was the opportunity. I arranged for treatment knowing that if it failed, it would not be from lack of effort on my part.

At the end of the first day of treatment and practice I felt that the technique did in fact give me control over my speech for the first time. The first nights during treatment were very restless, my subconscious perhaps refusing to admit what I already sensed. From the first day, I ceased to struggle against the vocal cord locks. I learned to recognize them and to respond with careful use of technique. I dedicated myself to using the technique correctly and at all times. The prescribed practice became my top priority when I returned home and began the follow-up phase of therapy. With the help of my family at home and an understanding supervisor at work, I was able to follow the program faithfully.

I still encountered occasional blocks in high-stress situations, invariably due to sloppy use of the technique. As my command of the technique grew, my confidence increased, and in situation by situation I was successful.

Word substitution was the first crutch I discarded. It took me a while to get used to always saying exactly what I originally intended to say.

By the fourth month of therapy, the phone was no longer an object of fear. I was now pleased to hear it ring, since it would present an opportunity to further practice my technique. The apprehension and former stress symptoms were gone.

By the sixth month, I knew that I could be completely successful if I kept at it. I had already been through some serious high-stress experiences with total fluency. I was having no problems with group situations, interviews, or phone calls.

The most difficult part has been to develop a high degree of concentration on the technique, regardless of my surroundings. Diligent practice and effort makes it possible. There were some early instances in which another speaker or questioner would become impatient for reply. I learned to not react to this, but to still take the second or so to employ the technique. It amazed me that no one ever realized that a flow was being employed unless I specially demonstrated it for them. Some people did indicate they thought I was speaking a little slower than usual.

I think I can best categorize the therapy as a learning process. I didn't become totally fluent overnight, but each day has increased the range of situations in which fluency is achieved, regardless of stress level.

At the age of thirty-five, I have started a new phase in my life. There are many things I have done during the last year which were quite beyond me before, simple things like ordering over the phone, calling the hospital in an emergency, inquiring about a new position, speaking easily to people—always a problem in the past.

I achieved a goal of teaching in my church, something I had long hoped to be able to do.

I changed jobs during the therapy, taking a position requiring constant interaction with people, under situations of considerable stress.

I have been able to eliminate the dependency I had on others to help me through situations, either voluntarily or by manipulation on my part. I feel that others can now count on me, and I can offer the kind of support and leadership I once shied away from.

———

To show that age is no barrier in overcoming the problem of stuttering, allow me, as a last example, to give you the case of a retired mechanical engineer—a man who stuttered for longer than most people live.

———

My case as a stutterer is unique in that I did nothing to correct it until I was seventy-four years of age. I stuttered mildly as a boy, but managed to get by without too much trouble. But after college, when I entered the business world, the situation worsened and I had my troubles. I attempted to speak freely, using human willpower, but the results were disastrous. I developed ways of getting by. I often coughed to get started; I avoided certain words, especially those starting with the letter s, and this resulted in very odd sentence structure. Sometimes my telephone conversations were most embarrassing. I did a very bad job of introducing others, asking for directions, and ordering in restaurants. At times I wanted to run and hide.

But I didn't. I struggled on, learning to live with a condition which was so abnormal. I often thought of seeking some sort of therapy but never did. Now I am just satisfied that I didn't, because, having talked recently with other stutterers who tried various curative systems (before Dr. Schwartz), I found that none of them were helpful.

I had a fairly successful business career in spite of my handicap, although I surely could have done better had my speech been normal.

Then, about twelve months ago I read an article in a Sunday supplement on stuttering, which described briefly a technique used by Dr. Schwartz and told about his book, *Stuttering Solved*. This intrigued me; I bought the book and started to read it. I attempted to use the technique described, in a halting way, and to my utter amazement it worked! Taking a sentence that would normally give me a lot of trouble, I found that despite my conviction that I would stutter, I didn't. I cried. I told my wife, and she cried. That was the beginning of freedom.

I soon became aware that applying what the book taught wouldn't be enough, so I wrote to Dr. Schwartz and arranged to join his workshop in San Francisco. That was about nine months ago. After a revealing two days at the workshop, there began the (sometimes arduous) work of mastering the technique under any circumstance that can befall a speaker. Frankly, I had no idea a wrong habit of speaking could be so stubborn. It seems so easy to master the technique under controlled conditions, but oh how easy it is to forget and return to the old habit. With the help of the weekly tapes reviewed by Dr. Schwartz's staff worker (bless her!), I am making slow but steady progress, and daily getting closer to the goal of complete correction of the old difficulty.

Proofs of progress are many. The automatic use of the technique is becoming stronger and stronger. Words starting with *s* give me practically no trouble. I use the telephone freely. I make introductions with ease. I order in restaurants for myself and others. I ask directions without difficulty. Speaking in public is becoming easier. I have given talks before more than a hundred people, and while not yet perfect, I have exhibited a freedom I never had before. I have not the slightest doubt my continued practice will bring about the elimination of the problem that plagued me so long.

To say that I am grateful is a complete understatement. When I recall the handicap I once had and note the freedom I now have, it seems like a miracle. And it is all so simple. I marvel at the perception Dr. Schwartz had developing the technique and its application. It promises a wonderful boon to countless individuals who are now in bondage to this awful affliction.

Finally I want to express my deep appreciation for the dedication of Dr. Schwartz and his staff in their wonderful work of helping stutterers. One feels the sincerity of their work and is aware of their strong desire to help through patience, encouragement, and scolding when necessary. They deserve strong praise.

———

These three speeches, given at various times and various locations, are testimonials to the perseverance of individuals who stutter. As you may surmise, the work is not easy. It is fraught with frustration, and the initial fluency can be misleading. But with all of this, something else emerges as well: And that is that there is a reward for hard work and that the problem of stuttering can definitely be conquered with sound technique, diligent application, and a good external support system.

5

The National Center
for Stuttering

The publication of my first book in 1976 brought thousands of responses as stutterers came forth to indicate that they had been deeply moved by its contents. Many felt I was describing them so accurately that they wondered if I was, or had been, a stutterer. All of them wanted treatment.

I soon recognized that alone I was powerless to meet their demand for treatment, a demand that was beginning to lay siege to my available time. I had been trained as a researcher and now found myself being forced into the role of clinician.

Furthermore, speech therapists were reading the book and beginning to contact me seeking training. I indicated that training programs would begin shortly but really had no concrete plan for implementing such training.

I expressed my frustration to a colleague who suggested that I develop an organization that would perform several functions. First, it would train speech clinicians. Second, and simultaneously, it would treat stutterers, the treatment being the initial process by which the clinicians would be trained. And third, the clinical material would serve as the basis for research to further improve the therapy.

And so in 1975 the National Center for Stuttering was born. It was funded by fees obtained from training clinicians and from the patient treatment program. The funds permitted the functions of the center to be supported on a continuous and self-sustaining basis.

Training

First we decided to focus the center's training efforts on public-school speech clinicians. Experience had shown that if therapy begins early, there is a better chance of effecting a good result.

The center has remained true to its initial focus and has maintained a continuing-education training program for public-school speech clinicians for more than a decade. Typically, the center trains one clinician from each school system, who then returns to that system to function as its resource person. In this way, a reasonably wide dissemination of technique is achieved.

Much work remains, however, since there are more than thirty thousand public-school speech clinicians in the United States. The center trains approximately seventy-five a year. It is hoped that in the future that number can be increased substantially.

Research

The center is also committed to continuing research. The vitamin and mineral recommendations and the food-testing procedure described in chapter 3 are examples of the results of the research program.

Parent Counseling

Another important function of the center is to advise parents if they see their child beginning to stutter. Here are the most commonly given suggestions:

- Eliminate all sources of refined sugar in the child's diet as much as possible.
- Provide a good multi-vitamin and -mineral supplement made expressly for children. Consult your pediatrician for guidance.
- Eliminate caffeine (present in cola and cocoa products, as well as coffee) from the child's diet.
- Eliminate all sources of stress in the child's environment as much as possible.
- Speak softly and slowly to the child and to each other in the presence of the child—especially slowing the first syllable.
- Allow the child plenty of time to speak, so that he does not feel the need to rush to get a word in edgewise.
- If the child is unaware of his speech dysfluencies, do not point them out. However, if the child is aware of the problem, suggest that he speak softly and slowly, particularly at the beginning of sentences.

Hotlines

The center maintains the National Stutterer's Hotline, a permanent toll-free 800 number, 800-221-2483, for any individual, or the family of any individual, who stutters, and the only phone number that stutterers can feel free to use to discuss their problems. A trained and sympathetic professional is available throughout the day. (In New York State, the permanent hotline number is 212-532-1460). Funding for these hotlines, including their staffing, is provided by fees obtained from the treatment-training programs.

All patients treated directly by the center have access to the NCS clinical staff through an almost twenty-four-hour telephone hotline. Stutterers are fragile at the beginning of their training and can easily recondition old fears. It is extremely comforting to know that a knowledgeable therapist is available almost around the clock to provide support and offer advice (all patients are given special telephone numbers for use after hours and on weekends).

Public Education

Informational lectures about stuttering are given to the general public as part of the center's program of continuing public education. The center also annually reviews the world's research on stuttering and presents it in an easy-to-read format for patients.

Support Groups

The center has organized dozens of support groups throughout the United States. It is safe to say that there is hardly a major city that does not have at least one club of air-flow users. The center is working to expand this network since evidence continues to show that individuals who are active participants in support groups can be expected, on the average, to make more rapid progress and to have an eventually higher rate of success than those that attempt to go it alone.

Certification and Training

Currently the center maintains a certification program. Certificates of Competence as Air-Flow Therapists are given to clinicians who demonstrate a basic understanding in the use of the techniques with patients. More recently, a Master Clinician status has been established. The Master Clinician's function is to train clinicians. This certification was begun in an attempt to decentralize a major function of the center through the use of a network of geographically dispersed instructors.

Much work remains, particularly in the area of providing services for the adult stutterer. Current research indicates that there are approximately two million such individuals in the United States. Training clinicians to work with adult stutterers is arduous and time-consuming. Adult stutterers can engage in subtle behaviors that often defeat the therapeutic attempts of beginning clinicians. It is safe to say that a period of at least one and a half years is required to train a therapist to work well with the variety of adult stuttering behaviors seen clinically.

Newsletter

The center has, for the past several years, published a quarterly newsletter. In it patients describe the results of their use of the air-flow and base-level-lowering techniques. In addition, useful pointers for increasing motivation and maximizing practice are shared.

Guidelines

Because of the time required to train a therapist, it is not surprising that a number of centers professing to use an air-flow technique do not. Here are some guidelines to use when selecting a program. First, ask whether a member of the staff has been certified by the National Center for Stuttering as an air-flow therapist. Second, ask to speak to patients who have been through the program to determine what their results have been. Third, ask whether or not the program provides a clearly delineated long-term follow-up support system. Fourth, take a dim view of any program that purports to effect permanent changes in a few weeks; it is absolutely unrealistic to expect that a lifelong problem will be changed so quickly. Fifth, determine whether the program considers the importance of base-level tension and its variability. And last, if any doubt exists about the competence of the program, call the center for an opinion.

There are so many different clinicians employing such a variety of approaches that it is often difficult to properly evaluate them all. But some definite conclusions can be drawn. Any program, if it is good, must produce an initial fluency quickly. If the technique does not accomplish this, the program should not be pursued. Similarly, stutterers should avoid the clinician who does not specialize in stuttering but instead treats a variety of speech or psychological problems. Stuttering is a specialized area, and its treatment is best left to those with extensive clinical experience. Nor should therapy be pursued if the clinician can offer no numerical probability of likely eventual success.

II

METAMORPHOSIS OF
A STUTTERER

by Dr. Grady L. Carter

Acknowledgments

I thank God. Without His grace I would have been unable to recognize the lessons stuttering had for me and unable to nurture the persistence necessary to maintain the quest.

I want to thank my wife, Devvy, who throughout my stuttering ordeal was the personification of love, patience, and support.

My thanks to Dr. Martin Schwartz for his efforts to clarify the cause of stuttering, and his development of the passive air-flow technique.

My gratitude to Carol Cohen for her invaluable assistance in the publication of this book.

I would like to thank Devereaux Carter and Bette Swanson, who were of incalculable value in the editing and typing of this manuscript.

I would be remiss if I neglected to thank Dr. M. Scott Peck and Richard Bach. These two have had a profound impact on my life, my consciousness, my striving to be the best I can be. I carry the gift of their wisdom with me daily.

Introduction

Stories about people overcoming handicaps wax poignant and sweet, with moments of deep defeat and wonderful triumph. Living through those peaks and valleys, however, is much more fluid and less defined. For me, overcoming stuttering was a crippling, agonizing struggle, a war littered with battles that first had to be recognized, then confronted and ultimately won. I won.

For most of my life I have said, "I wish I didn't stutter." I hoped against hope that some magical external force would descend upon me, sweep me up into fluency, and cast away the stuttering demon. Unfortunately I carried this childhood fantasy into adulthood. This fanciful delusion not only was unrealistic but also showed that I did not understand my own responsibility for my healing. It was not until I learned the passive air-flow technique that I realized that I had to make it happen—that I possessed the power all along to make that wish come true, by my conscious purposeful daily commitment to applying the technique to my speech.

There are no effortless miracle cures or simple solutions to the convoluted and complex syndrome that is stuttering. The journey through the stuttering maze to fluent speech required courage, determination, and independence of thought and action. These qualities are not mine alone, but are inherent in each of us.

My participation in this sojourn was at first hesitant and intermittent. For me to leave the negatively structured stuttering world in which I grew up and move into an awareness of a world where my only limitations were self-imposed, was frightening in its concept and awesome in its nature. Yet the more I positively participated in my life, the more effortless my application of the technique described in the book became. My stuttering atrophied from disuse and died a silent death.

Throughout my anguished thirty-three years of stuttering, I told myself that if I ever found a solution, a method of successfully dealing with my stuttering, I would take that message to other stutterers. I would let them know that they are not alone, that there are others who empathize with their pain because they have been there. I would assure them there is hope. In the spirit of encouragement and education, I offer my story. The personal examples I have included are to show the reader, and especially the stutterer, that a personal metamorphosis from stuttering can be accomplished. Anyone can do it—you need only give yourself permission.

DR. GRADY L. CARTER

Fort Worth, 1986

6

Reminiscences

As a child, I never knew myself not to stutter, not to suffer the fear, the tension, and the humiliation of stuttering.

In elementary school, we were all called upon to give oral recitations to the class. As I sat at my desk and watched the others take their turns, seemingly without effort, I could feel my body gradually tensing in anticipation. My hands would sweat. My body felt straightjacketed. My only thought was, I'm going to stutter, and they'll laugh at me. I tried with every ounce of my energy to suppress this thought, but the more I tried, the more anxious I became, and the more I stuttered. The humiliation of having to stand in front of the class, unable to communicate intelligibly, was so great that I was never able to finish my recitation. With my head bowed in shame, I would take my seat after each fiasco. The embarrassment and sense of defeat were overwhelming.

A teacher sympathetic to my plight encouraged me to attend school-sponsored speech therapy classes. During these sessions, an equally well intentioned but poorly equipped speech therapist had me parrot words that started with a particular sound on which I frequently stuttered. I then drew pictures of what these same words represented to me. The idea was to make me more and more at ease with these feared words, and therefore less afraid of using them. My stuttering was never directly confronted or even discussed. This activity served only to focus my attention more sharply on my stuttering.

I would return to my class after each session, my gaze glued to the floor. I just could not look up and see my classmates staring at me. I felt freakish and imagined that they felt the same way about me.

The six years of therapy were a waste of time and effort. I also had the dubious distinction of being the only student who had to leave class for therapy. I hated being different, but I was, because I stuttered.

I tried my best to hide this unwanted difference, to suppress it, to ignore it, and to at least appear the same as my friends. These vain attempts merely fueled my growing fear that people would discover I was "different," to the point where I became terrified to speak.

I was not aware that the fear and tension I had internalized was being "recycled," targeted to the muscles of my larynx. The more tense and apprehensive I became about my speaking, the more the muscles of my larynx unconsciously constricted, and the more severe were my laryngeal spasms, and hence, my stuttering.

It was in my early elementary-school years that I began to construct the image of myself as a powerless slave to my stuttering. I simply could not control it! My words came out twisted on themselves when I most wanted them to be smooth.

In the late spring of each year, all the sixth-grade classes in my elementary school came together to present a play delineating the history of our state. This "Texas Pageant" was the zenith of our six elementary-school years. It marked the end of our elementary-school career and the beginning of our junior-high-school career—a rite of passage to maturity.

Speaking parts in this series of historical vignettes were highly prized, awarded only to those students who had a history of making good grades in both academics and deportment, who showed leadership abilities, and of course, who spoke fluently. The day the parts were assigned I waited with hopeful anticipation. I really wanted a major role, and I felt I deserved to get one. Our teacher called me to her desk. My heart soared. I got a major part, I thought. It was not to be.

She said I would have received a major role in the play if it had not been for my stuttering, and that she did not want me to be embarrassed on stage in front of the whole school. On the surface this appeared to be a kind and thoughtful gesture, but on a more subtle level I felt she was telling me I should be ashamed of my dysfluency. I thought that since I presented myself to the world through my speech, if I should be ashamed of my speech, I should therefore be ashamed of myself. This experience helped contribute to the negative self-image I was beginning to construct.

When I stuttered my parents would say, in a disquieting tone, "Slow down, don't talk so fast." I knew my stuttering upset them. I felt their anxiety. No child wants to displease his parents and risk the loss of their love. From this fear sprang the origins of my secondary struggle behavior.

I began to develop tricks that would, at best, prevent a stutter, or at least shorten the duration and lessen the intensity of the stutter. To divert my attention from my stuttering, I hit my leg with my fist; I stamped my right foot; I shifted my weight from side to side, sometimes so rapidly I felt nauseated; I stood on one foot; I snapped my fingers; I bowed my head; I stood on tiptoes; I squeezed my eyes tightly closed—the list of tricks was lengthy and produced only temporary successes. After a few weeks the magical power of each trick seemed to wear off, and I was again entrenched in my stuttering.

As I moved into my junior-high-school years, my stuttering intensified. I had developed a bouncing type of stutter. My speech sounded like a machine gun as I repeated the first letter of the stuttered word. My new classmates took little pity on me and unmercifully kidded me about my stuttering.

As a result of one especially painful kidding session, I changed the pattern of my stuttering. I resolved that if I was going to stutter, I was going to do it silently. From that time, when I stuttered I locked my speaking mechanism, not uttering a sound until the word erupted in a sudden explosion.

The next therapeutic attempt urged by my parents was hypnotherapy. As a thirteen-year-old beginning my pubescent search for "who I was," I wondered if the fact that I could not talk right meant I was crazy. Did my parents think there was something wrong with my mind? Similar thoughts had occurred to me many times before, and I was willing to try anything—even hypnosis.

I proved to be a willing subject. After a very few sessions the doctor needed only to count from one to ten and I was at a placid hypnotic level. I remember being aware of such profound generalized muscular relaxation that I was unable to lift my arm from my lap. There was no fear of speaking while hypnotized, no outside tensions for me to recycle through my larynx. As I talked to my doctor, I felt for the first time in my life what it was like to communicate with another person in a relaxed manner. There was no tension in my neck, chest, shoulders, or abdomen. This feeling was absolutely delightful. Unfortunately, the ecstasy was short-lived. I found that once awakened from a hypnotic state, there was no carry-over into the "real" world.

In an effort to provide fluent speech in my daily life, my doctor gave me a posthypnotic suggestion. While I was under hypnosis, he told me that any time I felt I was going to stutter, I would rub the fingers of my right hand together. This diversionary tactic was meant to switch the focus of my tension from my throat to my hand, but the distraction worked for only a few weeks. My stuttering returned as rampant as ever and continued at that rate through the eight months I spent in hypnotherapy. The hypnosis was discontinued, notable only for its lack of success.

Never during this therapeutic excursion did I believe hypnosis would work for me. I saw it as dealing with the symptom of stuttering rather than with that mysterious causative factor inside me that "made" me stutter, a causative factor I knew was there but could not yet identify.

I hated my stuttering and myself when I stuttered. I resented being controlled by it. I would wrap myself in contortions of secondary struggle behavior in a futile attempt to push my words through my block. In my early high-school years I became so frustrated with the lack of treatment success, I began to believe I would never stop stuttering. In desperation, I changed my approach and began to adapt myself accordingly.

My tenth-grade English teacher announced one day that in order to pass her course each student must memorize, and recite in class, one hundred lines of poetry. I was not proud of an open admission of cowardice, but I simply explained to her that I would rather fail English than stand in front of my class and stutter through this assignment. Amazingly enough this ultimatum worked. She allowed me to write the memorized poetry instead of reciting it. Through the success of this avoidance maneuver, my fear of facing difficult speaking situations increased while my strength of character diminished.

I had become powerfully weak. My manipulation of people was not confined just to my schoolteachers; it permeated all aspects of my life. If a situation arose necessitating introductions, I let others who were fluent take the responsibility of introducing me. My stuttering made some of my friends a little uncomfortable, and I knew they would go ahead and introduce me if for no other reason than to keep themselves at ease. When I had to make telephone calls that I knew would be especially difficult, I cajoled members of my family into making them for me by playing on their sympathies until they acquiesced. My friends and family may have thought they were doing me a favor, but their help only served to fuel my manipulative avoidance of stuttering situations.

There were times when I could tell that my stuttering really irritated my listener, and if I did not particularly like the person I would exaggerate my stuttering just to make him feel more uneasy. This passive-aggressive manipulative tactic hurt me more than it did my listener.

While in school, if I had a question I needed to ask one of my teachers, I would whisper it to a friend sitting nearby. He in turn would ask the teacher my question for me. I was willing to accept the teacher's scolding for what she thought was inappropriate talking rather than muster the courage to confront her with the real reason I was talking in class without permission. I was too embarrassed to stutter in front of the class.

My manipulation antics even permeated my social life. In lieu of what I thought would be certain rejection if I stuttered through inviting a girl on a date, I convinced friends to do the asking for me. Luckily, there always seemed to be someone who was willing to take that burden from me. It was interesting that I was more concerned about my stuttering while asking for the date than while with the date. I rationalized that once she accepted my invitation she had chosen to be with me, stuttering and all, at least for one evening.

I remember one dinner date in particular when I really wanted to impress my date. I was so sure I would stutter when I tried to order, I told my date I could not make up my mind what I wanted to eat, and for her to go ahead and order. As soon as she had finished ordering, I looked up at the waiter and said, "Me, too." The possibility of my not liking what she had chosen was of little concern. I wanted only to avoid the stuttering pain and embarrassment.

Life was not always so simple, nor were problematic situations so easily avoided. The years passed slowly, and I found myself more than ever a forlorn inmate in the puzzling, debilitating prison of stuttering. At one point my parents thought that I would not stutter if my tension could be alleviated. They asked our family physician to prescribe mild tranquilizers for me. The tragic, yet almost laughable result was that I still stuttered, only a bit more slowly. The drugs, needless to say, were discontinued after a short time.

On more than a few occasions, I played the role of the dependent petulant child by purposefully stuttering more severely than usual in order to get extra sympathy and attention. There was always someone around me willing to coddle me, to try to compensate for my pain. For this reason, when it was time for me to go to college, I chose to go to a local university and continue living at home.

I began to grow more concerned about the elimination of my stuttering. I was rapidly approaching adulthood and grew increasingly uneasy because I continued to see myself as a stuttering child. The time had come, I knew, for me to take command of my own life, yet it seemed for every step forward I took toward autonomy and self-confidence, I slipped back two steps as I allowed my stuttering to make me feel like the child I once had been.

During my freshman year at college, I decided I would like to become a commercial airlines pilot. I visited several flying schools, but they would not accept me as a student because I stuttered. My chances looked bleak until I finally found a school willing to take me despite my stuttering.

Radio conversation with a control tower in routine and emergency situations is a crucial part of flying. At the airport where I trained, the air-traffic controllers came to recognize both my aircraft and my stuttering problem. In misdirected generosity, these controllers, by initiating any necessary instructions or clearances, relieved me of the task of talking to them. I readily accepted their help. It was an easy out for me, another way not to confront my stuttering.

An extended cross-country journey during the course of my

flight training was required. I was concerned about talking on the radio to air-traffic controllers who did not know me, but I rationalized my worries away with, "I'll be okay. I'll do fine." When I attempted normal radio contact with the air-traffic controller at the terminal airport near my destination, I found I was struck with a paralyzing block so severe I could not speak to these strangers. I simply could not utter a word. I was terrified. I wanted to return to the airport from which I had begun my journey, but there was not enough fuel. I had to land.

Without radio contact, my only option was a nonradio approach to the airport. I knew this would, at the very least, disrupt the smooth flow of air traffic at the airport and, at the worst, would greatly increase the chances of having a collision with another aircraft. But I really felt I had no choice. I made my approach, landed, and taxied to the ramp. My hands were clammy, my stomach was tied in knots.

As I looked up, I saw a man running toward me, screaming and waving his fist. He was one of the air-traffic controllers, and he was not very pleased with what I had just done. I stood for five minutes as he raved on and on about how I had disrupted coordinated air-traffic flow at his airport, and how lucky I was not to have had a midair collision, killing myself or someone else. I could not have agreed with him more. He asked if I had a radio. I nodded yes. He asked why in the world I had not used it. I somehow stuttered a reply that my radio was broken. He demanded that I get it fixed before I flew again, and I gestured that I would. As he stormed away, he was still admonishing me for flying an aircraft with a broken radio. My desire to conceal my stuttering had been all-prevailing.

After completing the remaining requirements for my private pilot's license, I applied to several commercial airlines, but each insisted I seek flight experience with the air force first. My application to the air force ROTC program at college was denied. The reason: I stuttered. Faced with what seemed to be an insurmountable obstacle, I abandoned my dream of becoming a commercial airlines pilot. Unfortunately, relinquishing goals, quests, dreams, and hopes is a typical behavior pattern for many stutterers.

Shortly after this rejection I changed my college major to premedical studies. One of my professors took an interest in me and my debilitation, and told me about the wife of one of his colleagues. He thought she might be able to help me since she had a graduate degree in speech therapy. My parents encouraged me to pursue this new hope, and once again I returned to conventional speech therapy.

During the following year I learned certain desensitization techniques: use of a metronome, delayed auditory feedback, white noise, "waiting out" a block, "easy" stuttering, and making myself stutter.

A metronome is a very small, battery-operated device, similar to a hearing aid, that is attached to a stutterer's ear. It produces a series of beats at consistant intervals. On the premise that a stutterer does not stutter when he sings, the inventors felt that stuttering resulted from the lack of speech rhythm. The rate of the beat of the metronome can be adjusted to impose an artificial rhythm or cadence on a stutterer's speech. In my case, the use of a metronome initially worked for several days, slowing my speech to coincide with the rhythm produced by the metronome and decreasing the frequency of my stuttering blocks. Gradually the diversion of using this device wore off and my stuttering returned.

Delayed auditory feedback dictated that I wear earphones cutting out all outside noise, and that I speak into a microphone. The rationale behind this device was that stuttering is reinforced as the stutterer hears himself stutter. What I said was fed back to me through my earphones at a delay that could be adjusted to between a quarter of a second and three seconds. This attempt to break the speech-hearing cycle proved to be impractical, not only because it was too cumbersome to be used outside the clinician's office but also because it prevented me from hearing other sounds.

The logic behind white noise followed the same line of reasoning: if the stutterer could not hear himself speak, he would not stutter. A nondescript monotone, fed through a set of earphones, prevented me from hearing anything I said. But I still stuttered. Even if it had worked, wearing the earphones during my regular daily activities was impractical.

The more nervous I became, the stronger my struggle behavior became. My speech therapist thought I might benefit from some behavior modification exercises. She said that to allow myself to block on a word was to reinforce the stuttering block itself. So she gave me reading exercises to do in which I would "wait out" the block. That is, I would not say the difficult word until I knew I could say it smoothly. Some of those pauses seemed interminable, although in a matter of usually no more than thirty seconds I would be able to say the feared word without stuttering. This was painful enough, but when I had two or three or more feared words linked together in a sentence, the waiting stretched into what seemed to be an eternity. After several months at this arduous task, I was able to read aloud simple short paragraphs without dysfluency.

In practical application, however, when I paused to "wait out" the stutter, people would think I was through talking, and often begin a new topic of conversation. This made me feel ridiculous and verbally abandoned. I realized this socially unacceptable pause was merely a substitution of one abnormal way of speaking for another. It did not take me long to discard this therapeutic maneuver.

"Easy" stuttering proved to be equally ineffective. My therapist sat me down one day and said, "Listen, since you're going to stutter anyway, why don't you make it easier on yourself?" Her logic sounded appealing, so I gave it a try. I was instructed to make a soft, easy, bouncing type of sound on the first part of the feared word. This was to allow me to glide into the feared word instead of assaulting it. This sounded good in theory, and was successful in the therapist's office, but not so in the real world. When I tried it in conversation my secondary struggle behavior was less violent, but I sounded like Porky Pig. There was plenty of laughter from those who heard me, laughter that hurt so deeply I think only those who have stuttered can possibly understand how I felt. A fluent person could never know how incredibly painful it is to try with all your being not to stutter, yet to stutter and be the brunt of laughter.

The most effective treatment I received up to this point in my life was based on the concept of making myself stutter. Its validity lies in the fact that it deals specifically with the fear of stuttering, rather than with the physical symptom of stuttering. It was through this approach that I first began to really look at the psychological interplay between my handicap and me. The first time my speech therapist announced that she wanted me to make myself stutter, I was not only reluctant but skeptical as well. It sounded non-therapeutic to me. But to my surprise it turned out to be amazingly effective.

As I sat in her office and read the paragraph assigned to me, stuttering every four words whether they were feared words or not, the tension I felt about my stuttering vanished. It was truly astounding. Confronting the stuttering, I was acting as if I had power over it; and I did, in the context that I made it happen instead of waiting to be attacked by it. In a sense it was okay to stutter when I initiated it, because I made the decision. I was powerful then. I had control of my speaking life for the first time.

I took this new therapy home with me. In the beginning, the blocks I initiated would slip from being controlled and self-initiated into being uncontrolled and involuntary. But after making myself stutter for about an hour, I reached the point where my stuttering was of my own volition. After twenty years of learning to hide my stuttering, now I was forcing myself to stutter. Taking this therapeutic tool out into the world, talking to people face-to-face, was the most difficult thing I had ever done. Miraculously, within a few weeks of grueling, concentrated personal effort, I appeared to have achieved total fluency.

The change in my speech was so abrupt that my speech therapist was astonished. As a test of my newly found fluency, she asked me to speak to a class of senior students majoring in speech therapy at Texas Christian University. She wanted me to tell them about stuttering from a stutterer's point of view. I was petrified, but at her insistence I agreed.

Time for the speech arrived. In the hall outside the lecture room, I told my speech therapist that I was afraid I would stutter. In fact, I knew I would. She said, "That's what they want to hear and it's okay if you do. But the surest way for you not to stutter is for you to open your talk demonstrating how you can make yourself stutter. In this way you will show them the power a stutterer has to desensitize himself to his fear of stuttering." She was right. The minute I made myself stutter on the first few sentences my tension evaporated. For the remainder of the speech I easily moved in and out of my stuttering whenever I wished. When I finished I was very proud of myself and my confidence soared.

Ten months into this latest program came the acid test, of critical importance to my life. It was time to be interviewed for medical school. I believed that no medical school would matriculate a student who stuttered through an interview. The desensitization techniques I had learned were put to use. As I went through my daily activities, I made myself stutter, studying people's reactions like a casual observer. The dim, fragile realization gradually emerged in me that most people did not seem to be concerned about the way I spoke. It was I who cared so deeply about my stuttering. It was I who was concerned about whether people would think I was bright or dull, witty or stupid. It was I who worried whether people would like me if I stuttered.

On the flight to my interview at a Midwestern medical school, I began to tense in anticipation. What if I stuttered? My first impulse was to fall back into the habitual pattern of not confronting my speech dysfluency. But as I pondered the dilemma, I decided I was not going to take the coward's way out. I would openly tell the interview committee that I was a stutterer, but that lately I had had remarkable success in my concentrated effort to overcome my problem.

And so it happened during my interview. Just as it had when I spoke before the class of speech therapists and admitted my dysfluency, my tension dissipated. I spoke smoothly, with a tongue as articulate and flowing as any politician's. I was elated. I returned home more excited about my victorious confrontation with my stuttering than about my successful interview.

Within a month I received notification of acceptance to medical school. I was overwhelmed with accolades from my parents, professors, friends, and neighbors about my acceptance but also about my not stuttering any longer. I began to believe I had performed some sort of miracle. I shifted my focus from that of an ongoing confrontation with my stuttering to that of basking in the self-indulgent glow of what I had accomplished.

It was not long before I began to think, Oh, no! What if my stuttering comes back? I'll disappoint all these people. They won't like me anymore. This fear and anxiety grew daily. I did not understand what I had done to gain this new-found fluency. And so, I knew if the fluency ceased, I had no way, no method, of regaining it. I did not realize that the seed of the healing was in my open admission to the world that I stuttered. That humbling confession was the mechanism that broke the fear-and-tension cycle of stuttering. Once there was no anxiety targeted at my larynx, there was no stuttering.

I was accepted into medical school, and to all appearances it seemed I had whipped the "bad guy," the demon that had made me different. For a change, my future certainly looked bright. But my lack of continued confrontation with my stuttering did me in. One day, like a nightmare come true, my stuttering returned with all its intensity. The miracle was over.

Graduation from college and my first year of medical school passed slowly and painfully. Fluency, the simple ability to speak without the embarrassing fanfare of stuttering, had tasted so sweet during its fleeting appearance. I missed it and longed to enjoy it again. I retreated into that familiar, self-imposed prison with stuttering as the guard at my cell door. This withdrawal was the best way I knew to keep a low profile and protect myself from any close scrutiny by the medical school. I was afraid if they found out I had started stuttering again, I would be expelled.

So I sat in the center of the classroom hoping I would blend into the crowd. I would not raise my hand to answer questions, even if I knew the answer. As soon as the schoolday was over I immediately left the campus so I would not accidently encounter anyone from the faculty or administration. I never attended student-faculty social gatherings.

During the summer break between my freshman and sophomore years in medical school I applied for my first hospital-based job, that of a surgical orderly. In the interview portion of my application, I was asked if my stuttering would interfere with any emergency situations I might encounter while at the hospital. I said I did not think it would. The director of personnel believed me, and all other things being in order, I got the job. There was just one hitch. No one in personnel had thought to let the nurses on the floor know that I stuttered.

My first morning on the ward I walked to the nurses' station to introduce myself to the head nurse. I stuttered badly. My face turned red, the veins in my neck bulged, my eyes closed, and my head bent over in secondary struggle behavior as I tried to break the block. Unfortunately, the head nurse did not realize what was happening and overreacted. Before I knew it, she had pushed me to the floor, and, as two other nurses pinned my arms and legs down, she tried to force a plastic airway down my throat. I was terrified. In fact, I was so scared that I screamed, without stuttering, "Wait a minute!" I was able to explain that I was a stutterer, and was just having a block on my name. They helped me up, apologized profusely, and told me they had thought I was going into epileptic seizure. We had a good laugh about it, but inwardly I was deeply embarrassed, hurt, and very angry at myself. In a cowardly but effective attempt to avoid similar situations, I put a name tag on my uniform. When people wanted to know my name, I simply pointed to it.

The energy and ingenuity expended by stutterers to avoid the pain and humiliation of the stuttering cycle is extraordinary. Further, the diverse network of evasive actions is just about as individualized as fingerprints. We stutterers mold our lives around methods of minimizing the anguish of stuttering: jobs requiring no oral presentations, spouses who speak for us, leisure time based on solitary activities. The mania of speech avoidance is one of the major directing forces, if not *the* major directing force, of a stutterer's life. My name tag was just one example of many such evasive behaviors in my own life.

Early in my second year of medical school, one of my psychiatry professors told me he thought he could help me to stop stuttering. We spent months discussing the feelings I had concerning my stuttering, never directly developing a treatment for the physical dysfluency but rather centering our attention on inner conflicts common to most stutterers: fear, frustration, and anger.

I felt the fear of nonacceptance. I saw myself as different, and in that difference not acceptable to people, not worthy of being given a chance to prove myself. In truth, I was projecting my own rejection of myself onto other people.

The frustration I felt was ongoing. I knew I was intelligent, but when others talked for me, my intelligence was hidden. The me who was projected to the world was filtered through those who talked for me. I was capable, but how could others recognize this?

I could not do so much as communicate a simple, short sentence without taking a horrendous length of time.

The anger I felt stemmed from the frustration. I was furious at myself for stuttering, and for taking the cowardly way out. I avoided speaking situations in restaurants, on the phone, and at social gatherings. I felt anger when someone ridiculed or mocked me, but the anger was directed more at myself than at the offending person.

The nine months I spent working with the psychiatry professor were very constructive. Although not completely resolved, these personal obstacles and tensions were at least clearly identified. However, my stuttering continued unabated.

During my junior and senior years of medical school, some of my clinical rotation responsibilities included taking medical histories and performing physical examinations. The physical exams were no problem, but it took me at least an hour to complete the detailed questioning involved in surveying the organ systems. Normally this takes ten to fifteen minutes. My stuttering was so intense and blocks so frequent that by the end of the history-taking both the patient and I were exhausted.

After a few of these marathon sessions, I formulated yet another avoidance mechanism. I spent an entire weekend sitting at my desk, typing a detailed medical questionnaire. I made several copies and gave one to each of my patients to complete. I felt guilty about burdening them with a task I should have done, but the pain of stuttering through each question was much greater than any guilt I felt.

An internship in the air force followed my graduation from medical school. During my stint in the general surgery service, each intern was assigned a patient to "present" to a nationally recognized physician serving as a consultant in surgery to the air force. I was to present my patient to Dr. Alton Ochsner, founder of the Ochsner Clinic in New Orleans. I had always had a great deal of trouble talking to people I regarded as authority figures, and Dr. Ochsner certainly qualified as one. For the week preceding his arrival I tried to think of any excuse to get out of my presentation of a patient. Neither my senior surgical resident nor my attending staff had any sympathy for me. I was going to present a patient to Dr. Ochsner and that was that.

The moment finally arrived. There I was, standing before Dr. Ochsner, my attending staff, senior and junior surgical residents, and most of my intern class. I was scared to death. I mustered all the courage I had and began to talk. The situation must have frightened the stutter out of me, because the first several sentences were the essence of smooth, uninterrupted, fluent speech. Boy, I thought, I've got this made. But just as I relaxed my guard and ceased to mentally confront my stuttering, *bam!* I produced a stuttering block the likes of which the world had never seen.

From there, my speech went so rapidly downhill that the patient, taking great pity on me, I suppose, began to explain his own disease to Dr. Ochsner. Words are inadequate to describe the embarrassment and humiliation I felt as I awkwardly tried to regain control of my presentation.

The rest of my internship and three more years in the air force passed before I once again engaged in any therapeutic approach to my stuttering. During my anesthesiology residency, a physiologist with a Ph.D., whose father had been a master acupuncturist in China, suggested that acupuncture might effect a cure of my stuttering. At his insistence, I submitted to four months of thirty-minute acupuncture treatments three times a week. I must admit that while the needles were in place they were so painful I did not stutter. After withdrawal of the needles, however, my stutter was still with me. Again, four months of suffering were to no avail.

"I wish I didn't stutter." For almost thirty years this had been my lament. I would fall asleep at night with that wish on my mind, and awaken in the morning hoping that somehow a miracle had occurred while I slept, that I would be able to speak the first words of the day, and all those that followed, with an untwisted tongue. Yet that unspoken hope merely led to a greater, more painful disappointment as my first utterances tumbled out in their familiar gnarl. The miracle simply did not happen. With growing despair, I settled into the sameness of my stuttering, knowing it would be with me day after day. Unfortunately, no matter how uncomfortable or unhappy I was, only when the pain of staying the same became greater than the pain of change did I begin to alter my life.

A requirement for completion of my anesthesiology residency was writing a research paper and having it published. I knew of this requirement before I started the residency, but I did not think it would cause me any problem. At least I would not have to present my paper as a speech. I was wrong. After publication, my article was chosen as part of the scientific program at a national convention on anesthesia. When the chief of my anesthesia department told me how proud he was of me, and how pleased he was my article had been selected, I panicked: All the papers at this meeting are presented orally. I can't stand before hundreds of people and read my paper. I'll be too embarrassed. Anyway, I'll stutter so badly they won't understand what I'm saying.

Over the next several weeks, I went to each of the other residents in my anesthesia department, asking them to go to the meeting for me and read my paper. I almost had one of them convinced to do it when my chief called me into his office. "Grady, I hear you are trying to get someone else to read your paper at the meeting." Like a child caught with his hand in the cookie jar, I was mortified. What could I say?

"Yes," I answered, and went on to explain that I just could not give that paper before all those people at the meeting. My chief said, "It is your paper and you are going to give it, or you will not graduate from this residency."

Fury flashed through my mind. How dare he make me stutter in front of hundreds of people? Had he no sympathy for me? Obviously not. From that moment and through my presentation of the paper, I hated him.

For the three months preceding the meeting, I practiced giving the paper over and over again. By the time of the meeting, I had read that paper so many times I had the whole thing memorized.

The day of the presentation arrived, and even though I had committed the paper to memory, I was petrified. I sat in the auditorium awaiting my turn at the podium in such a state of tension that my hands trembled, my heart pounded, and cold sweat beaded on my brow.

When my turn came, I went to the podium, laid my paper down, riveted my eyes to it, and began to read. In my mind, the audience ceased to exist and I was alone reading aloud to myself. Shortly after, my ordeal was over. Not once had I stuttered. I could not believe it. I was jubilant.

Settling back into my seat in the auditorium, I felt as though I had just come through an emotional wringer. Sitting there, gathering my wits, I reflected on how I had distorted my thinking about this event over the last three months. The omnipresent fear produced an undercurrent of tension I had carried with me twenty-four hours a day. But somehow I was still alive and the world still turned. Nobody in the audience was even aware of the incredible traumatic drama that had been played out within me at that podium. No one else took any special notice. I had blown the importance of the situation way out of proportion. In retrospect I realized how wrong I had been to hold any malice toward my chief. He had done me a great service, forcing me to confront my worst fear.

Toward the end of my anesthesia residency, my parents gave me a book entitled *Stuttering Solved* by Dr. Martin Schwartz. I started reading the book, though, to be honest, my parents were more enthusiastic about it than I was. In fact, I actually read only the first half of the book, stopping before reading the "Treatment" section. Not wanting to be disappointed by another treatment failure, I closed the book and put it on the shelf to collect dust. Someday, I thought, I might go to New York and learn Dr. Schwartz's technique, but I am too busy right now.

I began my private practice of anesthesia in Fort Worth, Texas, and continued to stutter severely enough to cause great consternation to many of my patients.

One patient in particular stands out in my memory. When I saw him on postoperative rounds, he told me how pleased he was with the anesthesia I had administered, but that he had been so afraid of his surgery he had used me as a scapegoat. I asked him what he meant. He said that my dysfluent explanation of his upcoming anesthesia had really frightened him, and he thought, I'm not letting this guy put me to sleep. He can't even talk. What if he stutters and gives me the wrong drug? I could die! He told me that his concerns about me were just his way of venting anxiety. Nevertheless, I was certain this was not an isolated incident. How many other patients had I frightened? I was upset with myself not only for causing these patients needless worry, but also for projecting an image of which I was not proud.

Because of these feelings, I initiated a search for help to control my stuttering for the first time in my life. This was a significant turning point. Until then, I had always begun therapy at someone else's suggestion.

Once again, I engaged the speech therapist I had had while in college. As I returned to her office, I realized that in spite of the great changes and triumphs I had made personally and professionally, I remained a failure in my own eyes. I was still that same stuttering little boy.

During my therapy sessions I was totally fluent in every speaking exercise. But when I left the cloistered, clinical environment of the therapist's office, my stuttering emerged as strong and rampant as ever. I pursued this tack for ten months before terminating my therapy sessions. Once again, my hopes for gaining consistent fluency had been dashed.

One day about a year later, I had a break between operations at the hospital. To pass the time I went to the surgeons' lounge, where I came across a newspaper from a neighboring city. I had never before seen a newspaper from that particular city in the lounge, nor have I seen one since. Yet there it was, opened to an article about stuttering and Dr. Schwartz. Having read the first half of Dr. Schwartz's book, I was curious, so I picked up the paper and read the article. It talked about the great strides Dr. Schwartz had made at the National Center for Stuttering, and gave a toll-free telephone number to call for further information. It emphasized that a stutterer should not worry about making this phone call, because the person at the other end expected to hear a stutterer calling. I dialed the number and learned there was soon to be a workshop at the Driskel Hotel in Austin, Texas.

When I went home that evening I took Dr. Schwartz's book from the shelf with renewed interest. I read the entire book twice. His approach to stuttering and its treatment made sense to me. I was intrigued and decided to enroll in the next treatment workshop.

During the two months preceding the seminar, I explored my commitment to change by questioning my readiness to give up stuttering. Was this really an honest desire, or had I merely been paying lip service to the idea of giving it up all these years? I asked myself why, after all these different therapies, I still stuttered. Even though I professed to hate my stuttering, I still participated in it. Therefore, I rationalized, I must receive some gain from it.

As I thought about this, I began to see how I had learned to use my stuttering to personal advantage. I had coerced people into making telephone calls for me, into ordering my food in restaurants, and into asking questions for me. I rarely dealt with salespeople, made oral reports, or participated in anything of an unpleasant nature involving speaking. The sense of power I gained from my avoidance techniques and manipulation of others was understandably gratifying. Family and friends were always willing and able to take the burden of even minor conversations from me. Their love and concern helped me avoid my stuttering, but in the end it did me a great disservice by perpetuating and enhancing my fear of stuttering.

I perceived myself as a stutterer, first, last, and always a stutterer; not a viable, young, intelligent person who just happened to stutter at certain times. Never was there a moment when I did not dread the next spoken word. It was an incredibly difficult and amazingly destructive burden to carry every waking hour, day after day, year after year. And yet, carrying this burden, I found a certain degree of security. I had an identity, a place, a device that set me apart. People always remembered me, if for no other reason, because I stuttered. In a strangely disquieting way, my stuttering had become a companion whose company I would have to relinquish if I became fluent.

If I were to gain my fluency, I would no longer be the "me" I knew. Could I be comfortable with the new, fluent person I might become? Up to this point in my life, I had avoided introspective questions of this sort, but now I had to ask and cope with them. What if I did not become the silver-tongued orator, the glib, clever person I imagined? Would I rather discover the answer or remain a stutterer living in an imagined world of all I could become? As painful as stuttering was, would the metamorphosis to fluency be more painful, more disruptive to my life?

After much soul-searching, I decided to give it a genuinely honest try. With my resolve firmly in mind, I headed for the workshop.

7

The Workshop

On the morning the workshop was to begin, I awoke quite early. Too excited and anxious to go back to sleep, I gave in to anticipation of the day. I dressed, ate breakfast in record time, and was out the door on my way long before necessary. As a result, I arrived at the Driskel Hotel nearly half an hour early. Since I did not wish to appear too eager, I looked for some sort of diversion to occupy myself for that half-hour.

A shoeshine stand was just opening, so I sat down to have my shoes shined even though they hardly needed it. As the man polished and buffed, I drew into myself, wondering about what was to come. Could this new technique be the answer for me? Had I come to the end of my slavery to the stuttering master or would this be another dead end, wasted effort, one more disappointment? I could feel my anxiety level rise, my body tense, my throat close. Yet there remained a glimmer of hope, the possibility that, just maybe, I could overcome my stuttering with this technique. Whatever the price, however much I feared another letdown, I knew I had to give this a chance. My shoes shined, I walked to the meeting room and went in.

As I entered the room, Dr. Schwartz asked me that terrible question, the one that is so simple but so difficult to answer, the one most stutterers have the greatest trouble answering: "What is your name?"

Over the years, by word avoidance and substitution, I had learned to escape from some of the stuttering traps I saw coming. But how could I do this when asked my name? I couldn't. There was no word I could substitute for Grady or Carter. The specificity of an answer always threw me. Knowing I had to give an exact response to a question always created an incredible amount of tension. Another problem with my name was that both Grady and Carter start with a hard consonant sound that tends to increase muscle tension in the larynx, thus facilitating premature glottic closure, laryngeal spasm, and stuttering.

When Dr. Schwartz asked my name, I stuttered and sputtered through it before I sat down, painfully, shamefully wondering if this was, indeed, worth all the embarrassment and anxiety.

Looking around the conference table, I noticed that there were thirteen of us, ranging in age from the early teens to the mid-sixties. Each, I thought, must have a history of numerous unsuccessful attempts at other forms of speech therapy. It was obvious from their expressions that they shared my own anxious mixture of fear and hope.

To my right sat a vibrant, intelligent, sixty-five-year-old woman who had for years been a "closet" stutterer. In other words, she had mastered the ability to word-substitute so completely that when she realized she was going to block on a particular word, she simply replaced it with another word she knew she could say without stuttering. This ingenious avoidance maneuver may sound incredibly difficult and complicated, but she had become so adept at it that her own daughter had no idea her mother was a stutterer. I had employed this maneuver many times myself, although I had not honed it to such a perfected state.

To my left was a young boy who looked twelve years old. He seemed bright, eager, and attentive, an average child in all respects except that he, too, was a stutterer. As he stuttered through his name a pall fell over him. He sank into his chair with his eyes downcast, clearly wishing to be anywhere else in the world just then. His pain was shared by those around the table, for we had all known it many times ourselves.

Once we had introduced ourselves, Dr. Schwartz began the workshop with a general overview of the stuttering phenomenon. I sat there listening to him address a question I had posed to every professional who had tried to treat my stuttering: "What causes stuttering?" The answer I customarily received was "No one really knows." None of my therapists had been able to give me a single characteristic common to all stutterers. They could only offer conjecture about stuttering's genesis. One nebulous theory stated that there was a "short circuit" in the neuronal connections between a stutterer's brain and mouth. I dismissed this idea because I would have stuttered constantly if such a deficit existed. This was clearly not the case. I had never stuttered when talking to my pet, or with an imaginary friend, or to myself. My stuttering was a true social disease—I only stuttered when I was with other people.

The pieces of this supposedly unsolvable puzzle began to fit together as Dr. Schwartz explained that stuttering is a habitual speech pattern, developed in early childhood, that is caused by tension internalized and directed to the muscles of the larynx, ultimately causing a laryngeal spasm. These tensions would be relatively minor in an adult but are major to a child.

I remembered being a very small child, stumbling over my words as I tried to talk to my parents, hearing them say, "Don't stutter. You shouldn't talk that way. It's bad. Slow down and start over." I had tried with all my might not to stutter. I was so frightened of displeasing them and losing their love, I tried to hide my stuttering. The more I tried to hide it, the more I stuttered. As Dr. Schwartz talked, I realized I was still following that scenario, bringing childlike fear of rejection into my adult life. It was not until later, through independent study, that I realized the negative self-image I had constructed from childhood was the fuel that kept my habit going in adulthood.

After completing the overview of stuttering, Dr. Schwartz showed us the passive air-flow technique, and we began our practice. We each took turns speaking into a tape recorder. There was no lying to myself now. I could not hide the quality of my technique from the group either, because the tape was played back for everyone to hear. Dr. Schwartz worked with each of us, teaching us how to evaluate ourselves and each other constructively.

At first, it was difficult. Not the physical action of allowing air to flow passively through my vocal cords—that was easy. But mentally resisting the urge to push at my speech, to hurry my words, was extremely hard.

I learned to relax. If I caught myself tensing and preforming the next word, I made myself stop and begin the application of the technique again. The initiation of this self-discipline was very difficult at first, but worth it when I realized that, with practice, the old habit of tension could be replaced by a new habit of relaxation.

That first day, we learned that the passive air-flow technique is 100 percent successful in preventing stuttering, but only if the stutterer uses it. Dr. Schwartz said he would not allow any of us to continue to the second day of the workshop if we did not use the technique during the afternoon session. This requirement did not cause me concern, as I had committed myself totally to overcoming my stuttering, but there were other participants in the class who did not cooperate with Dr. Schwartz. Their money was refunded and they left the workshop.

As we left our meeting room at the close of the first day, we were instructed to go practice what we had learned, first alone and then with others. We were to look through any magazines we had handy and in simple sentences describe aloud the pictures we saw, applying the passive air-flow technique after every four words. First I did this exercise silently, concentrating on the repetitive application of the technique. After fifteen minutes, I continued the exercise aloud, recording a few minutes. At the end of the exercise, the tape was used as positive reinforcement when I heard myself use the technique perfectly and as an educational tool when I did not.

The next exercise was to have someone "toughen" me, so I asked my wife to help. She rapidly fired short questions at me while I tried to answer using the passive air-flow technique. The point of the exercise was not to let her verbal speed disrupt the slow, smooth application of the technique. A few minutes of this exercise was taped, and I listened to it for both education and positive reinforcement.

It was not especially difficult for me to apply the passive air-flow technique when I was alone or with my wife. I was under low stress at those times, so the smoothness of my speech was not particularly surprising and I must admit I was still skeptical. My fluency just seemed too good to be true. Wanting to give this new technique a more stringent test, I used it that evening to order my wife's dinner as well as my own. The technique worked: I did not stutter. For the first time in my life, it seemed I had found a relatively uncomplicated therapeutic technique I could apply to specifically difficult words, or to specifically difficult situations outside the confines of a therapist's office, and be stutter-free. I was excited, but could the technique stand the test of time?

I awoke the second morning pleased with the events and results of the preceding day. Eagerly I dressed and walked down to the hotel coffee shop, telling myself that this breakfast was not going to be limited to choices I could order without stuttering. I could enjoy any food I wanted to eat now that I was armed with my new technique. I'm sure the food was delicious, but all I remember was the elation I felt after I fluently ordered my breakfast.

Dr. Schwartz began the second day of the seminar with a most profound and irrefutable truth: "Stuttering can be a stumbling block or a stepping-stone. It depends on what *you* make of it!"

We were then given the button.

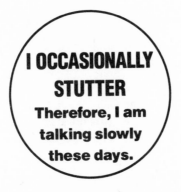

When Dr. Schwartz told us we had to wear that button, my initial reaction was "No way!" I had just started using a tool to get through my stuttering blocks with fluency, and I'd be damned if I was going to announce to the world that I was a stutterer, whether or not I blocked.

But my mind quickly flashed back to my senior year in college, when I attained fluency. When I openly admitted to my stuttering, it lost its power over me. Maybe this tack would be successful again. It was worth a try. As I made myself pin on that button, I began my rediscovery of the truth of Ralph Waldo Emerson's words: "Do the thing you fear and the death of [that] fear is certain."

So much of stuttering seems to revolve around fear. Since fears often lead to increased levels of tension, we were taught other ways of desensitizing ourselves to them. For instance, I was terrified of speaking on the telephone. For me, and I think for most other stutterers, the confrontation with a telephone must surely be the most ominous of all. As far as I was concerned, it was the single most devastating device ever invented, its specific purpose being to diabolically torture and torment me. Just looking at the instrument sent a chill to my core.

Could it be any other way for a stutterer? To be forced into a situation where the total perception of your being hinges on how you talk puts enormous pressure on you to hide the dysfluency, to suppress the stutter, to pretend it does not exist. Speaking into the telephone, you have no chance of camouflaging a dysfluency with a charming smile or a diverting gesture. Even writing down what you are trying to say cannot help. And therein lies the crux of the fear.

My fear of the telephone precipitated severe stuttering, which in turn further raised my anxiety level and resulted in even more laryngeal blocking. Dr. Schwartz led me through a hierarchy of desensitization steps designed to break this vicious cycle. For me, the key was to slowly and progressively gain mastery over my irrational fear.

The first step was to simply stand next to a telephone. I did this until I no longer felt any anxiety. I was allowed to proceed to the second step only when my anxiety had completely dissipated. Moving forward too quickly is a guarantee of failure in this desensitizing process.

The second step required me to pick up the telephone receiver and hold it in my hand. Again, I practiced this until I felt no anxiety: Next, I practiced dialing one number at a time until I could dial a complete phone number without any anxiety. These small steps, together with a number of others, were repeated until I was able to make a phone call to the information operator, asking for a specific phone number, without stuttering and without anxiety. It finally dawned on me that a telephone was just an inanimate object that could do me no harm.

The desensitization process is a slow, tedious, and demanding one. But if it is done properly, any irrational stuttering fear can be overcome. After a time, you can design your own desensitization steps to target specific problem areas, in effect becoming your own therapist.

Next on the day's agenda was a group excursion to the hotel

lobby. Dr. Schwartz arranged all of us in a circle and called us one by one into the center of the circle for our turn at "public speaking." Using the passive air-flow technique, we were to explain to the group who we were, where we lived, what we did for a living, and our thoughts about the technique.

Mine was the eighth name called, and by that time a group of curious passersby had gathered around our circle. There must have been thirty people waiting for me to start talking. It seemed like three hundred. As I stepped forward, my old fear of being laughed at returned. I overcame that fear by concentrating on my technique. Each application of technique during my speech made the next application easier. In fact, I was so fluent that I just wanted to keep talking. Dr. Schwartz had to ask me three times to give up center stage. Obviously, I was delighted with my performance, as were the others with theirs.

After returning to our meeting room we focused our attention on the various practice techniques Dr. Schwartz demonstrated. We learned how to record these practice techniques on audio tapes that were to be mailed weekly to the National Center for Stuttering.

Shortly before the close of the afternoon session, Dr. Schwartz explained that the consumption of certain foods and substances results in an increased level of tension in some individuals. These foods and substances, called "provocative" since they provoke tension, vary from person to person. For instance, it is commonly known that refined sugar can cause an increased tension level as well as increased activity in young children. In my own case, I found that tobacco was a provocative substance, nicotine being known to stimulate the central nervous system. I had smoked a pipe for a number of years, but had not realized that smoking actually contributed to my stuttering. It increased my base-level tension and thus made it more difficult to practice and apply my technique. Once I realized this connection, I gave up tobacco altogether.

8

The Metamorphosis

Before I knew it, the workshop was over and I was returning home. On the two-hundred-mile trip back to Fort Worth, I practiced constantly. This practice was both fatiguing and exhilarating. Fatiguing, because initially I had to put so much concentrated energy into the physical application of the technique; exhilarating, because I saw the frequency of my stuttering blocks decrease drastically.

When I got home that evening, I called my parents to tell them we had returned safely. I was totally fluent. I could feel their excitement over the telephone. They were amazed at how smooth and controlled my speech was.

Before I went to bed, I tried Dr. Schwartz's bathtub technique. This technique sounded simple enough at the workshop, but trying it that first time seemed more than a little strange. There I was, a grown man, lying in a candlelit bathroom, up to my chin in warm water, chanting "re-" as I inhaled and "-lax" as I exhaled. I have never felt sillier. After a few moments, though, I began to feel the tension I had internalized during the day drain from my body. At the end of the first twenty-minute session, I fell into bed for the most restful sleep I had enjoyed in years.

During my first full day at home after the workshop, Dr. Schwartz's refrain, "Use your passive air-flow technique when you don't need it, so when you do need it you'll have it," kept echoing in my mind. At first this application of technique was deliberate and strenuous. The temptation to go easy on myself was great, but I knew that doing so would perpetuate my dysfluency. Also, I had to guard against the temptation to become discouraged by one slip of technique. Instead of castigating myself for a single failure, I intentionally focused my attention on the times I successfully applied the technique. I made constant application of the passive air-flow technique my goal, and I became a zealot about practicing. The repetition of any activity not only makes that activity a habit but, once the habit is established, also perpetuates it. Through insight gained at Dr. Schwartz's workshop, I realized I was stuttering precisely because I had made a habit of doing the things that kept me stuttering: trying to hide it, not speaking for fear of its exposure, using word avoidance and substitution, and having others talk for me. I was not taking responsibility for my own speech.

I felt I would never overcome my malady if I performed, for only one hour a day, the activities that would break my stuttering habit, and performed, for the other twenty-three hours, activities that would reinforce it. By now I was totally committed. Realizing that my speech was my problem and not my monitor's, nor Dr. Schwartz's, nor my family's, nor anyone else's, I decided I needed to become my own motivator, my own mentor, my own monitor.

I constantly tested myself. The first test I created was to contact everyone at work: doctors, nurses, technicians, orderlies, secretaries—everyone. I showed them my stuttering button and told each of them I had learned a new speaking technique that effectively dealt with my stuttering. In fact, I wore my button constantly, on my labcoat at the hospital and on my street clothes. It brought lots of inquiries. I was amazed to see so many people interested in that button. "Hey, Grady, what does that button say?" "What's that button for?" "Let me read your button." "Where did you get your button?" "What's that button mean?"

When I heard these questions, I knew the people were "hooked." All my life, I had felt that the public in general had the upper hand with me when it came to speaking and conversation. Now, using the button as a device to broach the subject of stuttering and my passive air-flow technique to facilitate my speech, I felt I had the upper hand.

It began to make little difference to me whether people were interested in my speech. The important thing was that I was purposefully and publicly exposing myself as a stutterer. The open admission of my stuttering shifted the power from the stuttering to me. When there was nothing to hide, the fear was gone. When the fear was gone, there was no more stuttering. Through this catharsis I broke the artificial link between the manner of my speech and my self-worth.

I wore the button each day for six months. During this time it seemed I must have educated and demonstrated my technique to practically everyone I knew, and to many I did not know. I gradually lost my obsessive fear of stuttering and laid the button aside. I still wear it, however, from time to time just to keep my education and demonstration skills honed.

I made a contract with everyone at work. If any of them ever heard me stutter again, I would give them ten dollars for each stutter. I meant it too. A contract made without the intention of paying if I faltered was of no value to me. The contract still stands today, and I have yet to pay one person.

My success at the hospital was so exhilarating that I wanted my whole community to know about this breakthrough for the stutterer. I called the medical reporter for the largest newspaper in my city, the *Fort Worth Star-Telegram*. She was interested, and an interview was arranged.

She was polite and attentive as I described the stuttering phenomenon, using the passive air-flow technique. When I finished she said, "This is all very interesting, but do you know of any stutterers using this technique?" Joy surged within me as I told her of my dysfluent past. She found it hard to believe, but my co-workers soon convinced her I was telling the truth.

Following publication of the article, I received many telephone calls. It was surprising to me that so many people were interested in stuttering and the passive air-flow technique. I started thinking about getting this information to other doctors and organized a seminar, to be held at Texas Christian University, so that Dr. Schwartz could come to Ft. Worth and explain his techniques to the physician population. I managed to convince Harris Hospital–Methodist Fort Worth Medical Center (the hospital where I worked), Fort Worth Children's Hospital, and Cook Children's Hospital to co-sponsor the seminar with TCU and the Department of Speech Pathology.

Making requests of people had always been an almost impossible speaking situation for me. I organized this seminar to spread the word, so to speak, but just as importantly to test my passive air-flow technique. Could I make all those difficult requests for funding and facilities without stuttering? I did, and it was delightful. But the crowning achievement for me was when I was able to stand on a podium before five hundred people, give a relaxed, fluent welcoming speech, and introduce Dr. Schwartz. In my wildest imagination, I had never thought I would be able to do that.

A group of stutterers from Austin, Houston, and Dallas came to see Dr. Schwartz for a "refresher course" following the seminar. Most of them were doing a good job, but there were several people who, in spite of showing an outwardly willing nature, still stuttered badly. This was my first exposure to people who had completed Dr. Schwartz's workshop yet continued to stutter. Why did they continue to do so?

I talked at length to these stutterers and found that they all had one thing in common: they had not altered their self-image. They had not broken the negative, destructive thought cycle that dictated whether or not they would stutter on certain words or in certain situations. A forty-year-old engineer from Houston summed it up nicely: "Oh, I'll never stop stuttering, but the passive air-flow technique has decreased its severity, and that's enough." I resolved that this would not be my plight. My success was going to be complete.

I developed an insatiable appetite for books on taking control of one's own life, maintaining positive focus, and viewing personal problems as projects with opportunities for learning. I gradually became more aware of the responsibility I had to depend on myself. The major thrust of my attention now shifted from the physical application of the technique to changing my self-image.

Stuttering, I invariably thought of myself as a thirty-seven-year-old child who only cursorily participated in a world where everyone else could "talk right." Remaining withdrawn, seeking to avoid the pain of stuttering, I was willing to give others responsibility for my speaking. But in my efforts to avoid the pain, I only delayed it. Wherever I went, I would find people to talk for me, but that was no real solution to my problem. Each time I avoided a stuttered word or a stuttering situation, it became more difficult to face that word or situation the next time. My fear and dependency fed on each other and loomed larger as time went on.

It became incumbent on me, as with any stutterer who truly wishes to be rid of his twisted tongue, to scrutinize my interpersonal relationships, identifying those that were based on a stuttering dependency. Those dependencies had to be discarded, for they served only to impede the full realization of personal potential. Dissecting my environment I began to notice when friends would say "I'll make that telephone call for you" or "I'll explain what you want." I started refusing these offers. I no longer wanted or needed others to speak for me, because I now viewed speaking situations as opportunities for using my new tool, and for bolstering my new self-image.

Long static relationships began to change. This redefinition of roles was fostered by the self-confidence I gained as I saw the dominance of my stuttering dissipate. Some of those who had usurped my speaking responsibility probably had done so with the genuinely loving motive of sparing me pain. But there were others who consciously adopted the role of "rescuer of the stutterer," yet subconsciously did not want me to change. I gradually came to realize that some of these people gleaned a degree of satisfaction and gratification from my stuttering. It was through my dependence on their speaking for me that they found a part of their own self-worth. This dependence would undoubtedly be threatened if I overcame my stuttering. The recognition of this fact was the first difficult step to the achievement of my independence.

In *The Road Less Traveled,* Dr. M. Scott Peck capsulizes the pathology of dependence in a way that struck a nerve in me:

> In summary, dependence may appear to be love because it is a force that causes people to fiercely attach themselves to one another. But in actuality it is not love; it is a form of antilove. It has its genesis in a parental failure to love and it perpetuates the failure. It seeks to receive rather than to give. It nourishes infantilism rather than growth. It works to trap and constrict rather than to liberate. Ultimately it destroys rather than builds relationships, and it destroys rather than builds people.

I quickly found that those who truly loved me were unconditionally supportive of my efforts to change my speech and of my newly discovered independence. My wife as well as my parents committed themselves to creating an environment in which I was not only free to take responsibility for myself and my speech, but moreover, was encouraged to do so. They did not interpret this quest for separateness as a personal loss, but instead a fulfillment of our relationship and an affirmation of our shared love. It was by letting go that we all received. They shared in my triumphs and rejoiced with me.

Even though my stuttering was finally bested, I found that cultivating my new positive self-image was much more demanding than I had imagined. For me to leave the negatively restrictive world I was accustomed to and move to an awareness of a world where my only limitations were self-imposed was frightening in its concept and awesome in its nature.

My focus had been so negatively fixed that I would not allow myself to remember, or even to acknowledge, any compliments I received. I felt unworthy of even the most minute accolade. I had subconsciously built this negative self-image since early childhood. In its construction I selected only those experiences that would reinforce the vision of myself as a limited, confined, helpless dupe, a person powerless to break free from stuttering. I firmly believed that "They will not like me when they know I stutter." So I compromised myself by not saying what I really felt and by not living up to my potential. I never found what I sought: the approval of others and my internal peace.

Had I allowed my stuttering to be a justification for my negative self-image? Or had my negative self-image evolved into a self-fulfilling prophecy? Was I using this negative self-image to get sympathy, love, or attention? Had *I* really brought myself to such a dreadful place? As painful as a tooth extraction, the answer came: a resounding yes.

It was not until I began to link words fluently into sentences that I started to question my negative self-image. I wasn't so bad. I had the tendency to stutter, but that did not make me horrible or twisted or crazy. So what if people knew I stuttered? What could they do to me? The truth was, they could not do anything I didn't allow them to. People who were so narrow-minded that they based whether or not they liked me on the character of my speech, rather than on its content, were not worth the worry.

I realized that stuttering was more than just a physical problem and more than just a psychological problem. It was both. If I stuttered, I saw myself as a stutterer; if I saw myself as a stutterer,

I stuttered. One problem perpetuated the other.

Now I had a physical tool to prevent the manifestation of stuttering. I removed the thought that I would stutter on certain words, or with certain people, or in certain situations, from my mind. I stopped concentrating on what I was relinquishing and concentrated on what I was obtaining. I began to use creative visualization techniques to reinforce my new self-image, and I restructured my life to include two fifteen-minute sessions of quiet meditation and visualization each day. I saw myself as a relaxed, controlled person, confident in my use of the passive air-flow technique. I learned to project an image of myself onto a mental screen and would picture myself in various types of speaking situations, feeling no anxiety or tension. I imagined these scenes in such detail that I could feel I was actually living each experience. Meditation and visualization helped me convince my subconscious mind that I could control myself and my speech, no matter what the situation. Sustaining and strengthening these positive images was foremost in my mind. I realized that the way I thought of myself was going to be the way I manifested myself. All I had to do was give myself permission to use the creative power I had possessed all along. I had brought myself to where I was, and only I could extricate myself from the stuttering cycle.

I realized that I was free to do whatever I wanted, to stutter or not to stutter. No one else made me stutter—I allowed myself to stutter. I allowed certain people, situations, or words to affect me. It became clear that if I stuttered again it was because I chose not to use my new tool. This was hard to accept at first, but was nevertheless irrefutable.

9

Death
of a Friend

I do not remember the exact time, or even the day, but I was sure he was dead. Once I became fluent, one of the most reliable parameters that defined my self was gone. The complex, carefully constructed system that had served to differentiate me from other people and to define my role in various life situations had changed dramatically. This left me a little unsteady. Yet I was, at last, free to express outwardly the Grady I had suppressed for years.

When my friend, stuttering, went to his death—and he did as soon as I sent him—I was not sorry. I began to see that going through the long, painful process of overcoming stuttering had been a growth experience.

I learned that to reach within myself and grasp the best I can be is more than just a physical or intellectual act. It is more than just controlling emotions. It is, in truth, a spiritual act, a continuous process of becoming. To change from the consciousness of a stutterer, with all that that entails on both physical and emotional levels, to that of a nonstutterer, is to touch the bedrock of one's being.

I learned what it feels like to transcend oneself; to go beyond self-imposed limitations. I saw that for most of my life I had been using only a small fraction of my potential and had rationalized this behavior with one excuse after another, each making failure acceptable. I began to accept the uncertainties of my future with a sense of anticipation, knowing I could take my life wherever I chose.

You wish you did not stutter? You need never stutter again. You can win in the end. You can take the defeats and triumphs you have already lived through, and use the gifts each has brought you to refine your character and rejuvenate your courage. Instead of worrying about whether you are different, you can concentrate on being just what you want to be. You can make the decision that you are really ready to stop stuttering now. You can stop manipulating the people who love you and start depending on yourself, your own capabilities and talents. You can set yourself free from those who would, with all the best intentions, undermine you. You can shed all those tedious, warped excuses you have been using all this time to remain dependent. You can ignite the spark of your self-actualization by embracing commitment, work, and faith. Do not kid yourself for a moment into believing you have no choice. You do!

You can cease to participate in the stuttering cycle. You can replace your negative self-image as a stutterer with a positive concept of yourself as someone who has smooth, relaxed control of your speech. You will soon come to view the world as an intriguing arena where you can find innumerable opportunities to practice and improve your techniques. Self-pity will be replaced by self-confidence.

If you are a stutterer, when your friend dies, you might feel a sense of stark abandonment and sudden vulnerability coupled with heightened expectations of yourself that provoke anxiety. But you can develop a whole new relationship with yourself as a fluent, expressive individual. You have reached for this book and thereby have grasped the tool that can enable you to shatter the old stuttering cycle and build a new speaking life for your self, if you so choose.

You can gain mastery over that diabolical friend and let him die. Then the miracle will be *you.*

The following is a compilation of some of the many books that found their way to me as I struggled to learn the lessons stuttering offered. This list is included with the hope that those who choose to journey through these volumes may also find them helpful.

Bach, Richard. *Illusions.* New York: Delacorte Press, 1977.

———. *Jonathan Livingston Seagull.* New York: Macmillan Co., 1970.

Berne, Eric, M.D. *Games People Play.* New York: Ballantine Books, 1964.

Browne, Harry. *How I Found Freedom in an Unfree World.* New York: Avon Books, 1973.

Buscaglia, Leo, Ph.D. *Living, Loving & Learning.* Thorofare, N.J.: Charles B. Slack, 1982.

Gawain, Shakti. *Creative Visualization.* New York: Bantam Books, 1978.

Harris, Thomas A., M.D. *I'm OK–You're OK.* New York: Avon Books, 1967.

James, Muriel, Ed.D., and Jongeward, Dorothy, Ph.D. *Born to Win.* Reading, Mass.: Addison-Wesley Publishing Co., 1971.

Kopp, Sheldon B. *If You Meet the Buddha on the Road Kill Him.* Palo Alto, Calif.: Science and Behavior Books, 1972.

Lair, Jess, Ph.D. *"I Ain't Much, Baby—But I'm All I've Got."* New York: Fawcett Crest Books, 1969.

Maltz, Maxwell, M.D. *Psycho-Cybernetics.* Englewood Cliffs, N.J.: Prentice-Hall, 1960.

Olson, Dr. Ken. *The Art of Hanging Loose in an Uptight World.* New York: Fawcett Crest Books, 1975.

O'Neill, Nena, and O'Neill, George. *Shifting Gears.* New York: Avon Books, 1974.

Peck, M. Scott, Ph.D. *The Road Less Traveled.* New York: Simon & Schuster, 1978.

Roberts, Jane. *The Nature of Personal Reality: A Seth Book.* Englewood Cliffs, N.J.: Prentice-Hall, 1974.

Rogers, Carl R. *On Becoming a Person.* Boston: Houghton Mifflin Co., 1961.

Schuller, Robert H. *Tough Times Never Last, But Tough People Do!.* New York: Bantam Books, 1983.

Silva, Jose. *The Silva Mind-Control Method.* New York: Simon & Schuster, 1977.

Simonton, O. Carl, M.D. *Getting Well Again.* New York: Bantam Books, 1980.

Smith, Manuel J., Ph.D. *When I Say No, I Feel Guilty.* New York: Bantam Books, 1975.

Weinberg, Dr. George. *Self Creation.* New York: Avon Books, 1978.

Appendix A

A Study of the Long-Term Effects of a Multidimensional Treatment Program for Stutterers

The purpose of this study is to present data relevant to the long-term effects of the multidimensional treatment program described in this book. The results are based upon a population of 625 patients who participated in the two-year program.

Subjects. The experimental population was composed of 492 males (mean age, 31.6 years) and 133 females (mean age, 27.4). Almost all had had speech therapy or psychotherapy at some point in their lives prior to enrolling in the NCS program. For 538 patients, their overt struggle symptoms ranged from mild to severe; for 87 patients, there were no overt struggle behaviors, but rather a well-developed word-substitution capability. This group, labeled "closet stutterers," was comprised of 62 females and 25 males.

Method. Each patient was treated using the methods described in this book. All learned the techniques for subtracting speech tension as well as those for reducing base-level tension. They all received weekly individualized assignments and sent tape cassettes to their therapist at the center on an average of at least once each ten days for twenty-four months. All participated in the vitamin-and-mineral supplementation program and the provocative-food-assessment task. All were required to attend local club meetings or to communicate regularly by telephone with fellow patients in their area. All attended at least three regularly scheduled refresher courses during the twenty-four-month period.

Prior to and at the end of the two-year period the patients were called upon to complete a detailed questionnaire. The questionnaire was a self-assessment of relative percent speaking success in each of twelve representative speaking situations. Test–retest reliability of the perceptual judgments indicated high reliability. The test was also readministered after thirty-six months to determine the effects of a post-treatment year upon the groups' judgments of their performance.

Results. At the end of the initial twenty-four-month period, 96 percent of the patients reported that the program had been successful. One year after termination of therapy, at thirty-six months, the success rate had dropped to 93 percent.

Discussion. The definition of success used in this study was "to be essentially symptom-free in all daily routine speaking situations." There was no attempt to define success as total elimination of undesirable habits, but rather to define it in a functional sense—that is, to function routinely without stuttering, word or sound substituting, or avoiding speaking situations.

Might the patients slip once in a while and stutter? The answer is yes. But they could recover immediately and, most importantly, reported that they were not psychologically devastated by the block. They knew it was caused by a failure to employ technique and further knew they could take immediate action to prevent further blocks from occurring.

Thus the results of this study indicate that for adults, well over nine out of every ten can expect to have a relatively permanent success with the techniques described—provided that they are religious in their adherence to all aspects of the program.

But what of the "failures"? Some, interestingly, may not be. For example, one of the patients, a stockbroker, entered the program, performed well during the initial phase, followed that by entering a telephone hierarchy, spent an unusually long time going through the hierarchy (four months), practiced several other hierarchies to success and, at eighteen months, quit. When tested, both at twenty-four and thirty-six months, the patient was still stuttering in some situations but reported overall that he personally considered the program a success. He revealed that his major, if not sole, purpose in entering the program had been to become fluent on the telephone since, if fluent, he could call new customers and be expected to increase his income substantially. The excessive amount of time spent on the telephone hierarchy was, therefore, a reflection of his personal emphasis. His business had increased significantly and, although he was stuttering in a number of situations, he had achieved his major goal. The program had performed its function for him. It was a success.

Many patients, after improving substantially in a number of speaking situations, are quite content with their accomplishment and simply stop practicing. There may be several situations in which they have consistent difficulty, but these occur for them so infrequently or are so relatively unimportant that the motivation for continued practice is nonexistent. These individuals are pleased with their result but from our research point of view are considered part of the "nonsuccess" group.

The slippage of three percentage points between the twenty-four- and thirty-six-month assessment represented approximately twenty individuals who reported the reoccurrence of difficulty in some speaking situations. All 625 patients had been without formal therapy for a year, and it was surprising to find such a small number reporting difficulty. It was possible to reinitiate treatment for eleven of the patients and, after a month, all had recovered to their twenty-four month levels. These results suggest that some form of periodic refresher course may be required for a small group of patients for a period beyond the formal two years of practice.

One important additional result emerged from the study. The likelihood of relapse appears to be great in the first five months of treatment. The patients are fragile. A high-stress episode can provoke an onset of stuttering that, if left unchecked, can result in a disastrous downward spiral in performance. We have discovered that the support groups, hotlines, weekly monitorings, and refresher courses have saved dozens of patients from relapse. We are left with the inescapable conclusion that all treatment programs must provide these services if patients are to achieve comparable levels of success.

Appendix B

Foreign Workshops

Shortly after *Stuttering Solved* appeared, I received word that the foreign rights to my book had been sold to a number of publishers. Within two years, the book had been translated into French and German. A version had also appeared in Great Britain. I began to receive letters from stutterers in these countries, letters that contained the same plaintive requests for treatment.

Was there anyone trained in my method in London? Was I planning to visit Germany? Could they come to the United States? For the first several years my response was that I was not prepared to visit Europe, but if they wished treatment, they could travel to the United States and work with me at the center.

A number of individuals took advantage of the offer. And it wasn't long before I was seeing a steady stream of individuals from abroad. The workshops in French were facilitated by the fact that I am fluent in the language. But the situation for German was different. Here, for the first time, it was necessary to employ an interpreter. I discovered, however, that treatment in a language unknown to me was as effective as treatment in English.

In other words, I discovered that I had developed a universal treatment for stuttering; the peculiarities of a particular language were irrelevant. Passive breathing is passive breathing, and a first syllable is fast or slow regardless of the language. If there was evidence demonstrating that the technique treated the cause of stuttering, this independence from language appeared to be it.

In 1980 I had an opportunity to visit Japan. My book had not been translated into Japanese, and attempts to sell the rights to Japanese publishers had been unsuccessful. In spite of protestations to the contrary, Japanese publishers felt that their language was so different that my methods probably would be ineffective. I, of course, knew this to be untrue, since I had treated several Japanese successfully in New York through interpreters.

At my hotel in Tokyo I arranged with the concierge to spend an evening with a Japanese couple as a form of cultural exchange. A university student studying English would function as interpreter.

My hosts, in their early seventies, enjoyed receiving foreign visitors in their home. He was a retired manufacturer of kimonos, she, a former schoolteacher. She had stopped teaching with the birth of the first of her four children. During the course of the evening I asked her whether, as a schoolteacher, she had seen much stuttering in the classroom. The interpreter, for the first time, paused to take a dictionary from his pocket. The word *stuttering* was not part of his vocabulary. When the question had been translated, the woman indicated that she had indeed seen stutterers and that she had taken care of the problem using the ancient method.

What was the ancient method? I inquired. Her response was direct: "We lit a candle and placed it just in front of the child's mouth. The child was to breathe in through the mouth and then let some air out calmly so that the candle just barely flickered, and then he was to begin speaking softly and slowly."

Here was the air-flow technique, and although there was no mention of base-level tension, the users of the ancient method undoubtedly experienced some measure of success.

When I questioned her still further, her answer was abrupt. She said, "I have told you how we took care of the problem of stuttering. Can't we please now go on to something else?"

I had the opportunity to visit several Japanese speech pathologists who had obtained Ph.D.s in the United States after the war. I found them still using the outdated techniques of the fifties, and when I questioned them about the ancient method, they dismissed it summarily, saying it was merely one of a whole series of old approaches that had failed. When I inquired whether they had ever attempted to use it themselves, their answer was an emphatic no.

In 1982 I visited Germany to conduct the first of a series of workshops. Individuals came from all parts of the country to participate. The results were so successful that clubs have now been established in the country's major cities and word of the results has spread to Austria and the German-speaking portions of Switzerland.

I also demonstrated my technique in Africa and in the process discovered that the Zulu have a rather interesting attitude toward stuttering. They view it as a sign of wisdom and, as a matter of fact, if an individual acts in a way they perceive as wise, they call that individual "stutterer" in spite of the fact that he does not have the problem. I remember once treating a man from Zululand. He owned a large farm and related to me that when he told his Zulu farmhands that he was going to have his stuttering treated, they viewed him as mad since, to them, he was going to have a portion of his wisdom removed.

One of the most unusual venues for a workshop was in the small city of Whitehorse in the Yukon Territory. A woman had traveled from Whitehorse to Lake Tahoe to attend one of our workshops. (Her story is told on page 70.) After the workshop, she returned and engaged in a lengthy process of educating and demonstrating. Her speech became remarkably fluent. It soon became apparent to her that individuals were expressing an interest in being treated by me. I indicated that I would be willing to make the trip to Whitehorse to conduct a workshop provided that the local speech therapist would agree to be trained.

The attendees at the workshop were an unusual group. There was a fur trapper, a gold prospector, an oil-rig operator, the owner of an old, deserted inn on a distant mountain, and a truck driver. They had gathered for the workshop and were to return to their isolated circumstances as soon as it was over. I informed them that it would be necessary to talk to other people. This, they assured me, would be no problem since, although they were alone, they used their radios frequently as means of communication. Later I was to learn that for months after, the air waves in the territory crackled to the sounds of toughening and discussions of flutter and slowed first syllables.

Last is the story of the sheikh's son, and though it did not originally take place on foreign soil it did, in fact, later on, in a strange way. A forty-five-year-old son of an Iraqi sheikh, educated at the London School of Economics, possessed moderate stutter. His representative contacted me with a request that I see the man for an evaluation. The evaluation was to take place at his employer's apartment at the Waldorf Astoria Hotel in New York. Security reasons, I was told, prevented his highness from visiting me at the center. I agreed to the request, arrived at the hotel, and was ushered into a private elevator that brought me to the appropriate floor.

There I met the first of a series of bodyguards who, after a quick, but thorough, screening with a metal detector, led me into a small sitting room, where I made the acquaintance of his highness.

His English was impeccable and his stutter moderate. I evaluated him and took my leave. When contacted later by the representative, a rather interesting question was asked: "What would be the best possible treatment that could be arranged for his highness?" My response was that he be treated by me for two days and that he then work daily with a therapist who would treat him almost continuously.

I had in mind a speech therapist whom I had treated several years earlier for a stutter. His royal highness would not only benefit from continuous therapy, but the therapist himself would also be using the very technique that he was calling upon his patient to use.

His royal highness accepted the proposition. I contacted the therapist and arranged for him to observe a workshop before going off to be the "court" therapist. He was to spend six months at the task. He agreed since the financial remuneration was appropriate. After a few months, he became a personal assistant to his highness and has never returned. His highness' speech has been successfully treated and, in exchange, the profession has lost the services of a competent speech clinician!

In all countries of the world, when reliable statistical surveys have been conducted, results have shown that approximately one percent of the adult population stutters. This means that in India, for example, there are more than six million stutterers. The task of providing treatment for so many individuals is unthinkable. In the United States, there are two million so afflicted. The probability of intervening in a significant degree in this population, given its size, is also remote. The best we can hope for is that through a process of gradual training, sufficient numbers of therapists will be available so that those actively wishing to control their problem can receive the support and training necessary to do so.

Appendix C

Treatment-Training
Workshops

Each year a series of treatment-training workshops is conducted throughout the United States. In fourteen cities, therapists acquire their initial exposure to the air-flow technique by observing treatment administered either by myself or an associate from the center. A carefully selected heterogeneous group of patients is chosen. Heterogeneity permits the demonstration, to both patient and clinician, of the irrelevance of any concern for the type or severity of stuttering. Violent, overt stutterers sit across from closet stutterers. Prolongers confront repeaters. And all are treated in similar fashion, and for all the symptoms abort virtually immediately.

The cities in which these treatment-training workshops are conducted are: Atlanta, Boston, Chicago, Dallas, Denver, Houston, Los Angeles, New York, Philadelphia, Phoenix, San Francisco, Seattle, St. Louis, and Washington. Those wishing to be treated or trained at one of these workshops are encouraged to use the hotlines (800-221-2483; in New York: 212-532-1460) to contact the center for further information.